PRAISE FOR MOLLY'S STORY

"Terrific, charming and engaging! Molly tells her story in a way that makes the reader want to try new behaviors."

—Carolyn Robertson, Associate Director of the Mount Sinai Diabetes Center

● ◆ ●

"This book fills a real gap. People who have diabetes need something like this to help them understand what they are going through. The monkey is so cute that people of all ages will enjoy it!"

—Rick Mendosa, Medical Writer and Diabetes Consultant

● ◆ ●

"I sincerely believe that everyone concerned with diabetes can learn from this delightful book. **Molly's Story** *is up to date and accurate and should be particularly useful to the parents of children with newly diagnosed type 1 diabetes. While it explains the complexities of living with diabetes, it also instills the attitude of 'If Molly can do it, so can I.'"*

—Jere Goyan, FDA Commissioner (1979–1982)

● ◆ ●

"This is a charming and informative book. I think kids can see themselves in Molly, in her mischievousness and her ambivalence about her treatment regimen, and her willingness to try different foods and activities should inspire them."

—Rob Dinsmoor, Medical Writer Specializing in Dia

＊ ◆ ＊

"What a great idea for an educational book! I was impressed by the way the authors were able to make difficult issues easily understandable. The photographs and drawings assist wonderfully with the information and training that is so necessary for people with diabetes!"

—Dr. Jonathan RT Lakey, Director, Human Islet Isolation Laboratory, University of Alberta

＊ ◆ ＊

"Molly's Story takes essential concepts in diabetes and makes them accessible to young and old. The photos of Molly are charming and the humor is delightful. Molly's positive attitude is uplifting and her story proves that education can be enjoyable."

—Scott R. King, President, Islet Sheet Medical

＊ ◆ ＊

I Have Diabetes Too!
Molly's Story

CAMILLE R. DORIAN &
MOSHE SHIFRINE, PH.D.

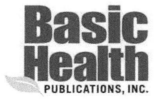

Basic Health
PUBLICATIONS, INC.

Basic Health Publications, Inc.

Library of Congress Cataloging-in-Publication Data

Dorian, Camille R., 1950–
  I have diabetes, too : Molly's story / Camille R. Dorian, Moshe Shifrine.
    p. cm.
  Summary: Information about the symptoms and treatment of Type 1 and Type 2 diabetes, along with discussion of exercise, eating plans, and more are presented from the perspective of Molly, a monkey with insulin-dependent diabetes.
  ISBN 978-1-59120-074-1 (Pbk.)
  ISBN 978-1-68162-904-9 (Hardcover.)

  1. Diabetes—Juvenile literature. [1. Diabetes.] I. Shifrine, Moshe. II. Title.

  RC660.5.S536   2003   2003004238
  616.4'62—dc21

Copyright © 2003 Camille R. Dorian and Moshe Shifrine, Ph.D.

Editor: Carol Rosenberg • Illustrations and photographs: Camille Dorian
Typesetter: Gary A. Rosenberg • Cover design: Mike Stromberg

Contents

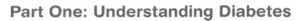

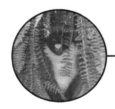

Part Three: Diabetes in Depth

Part Four: The Glycemic Index

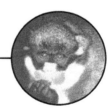

Part Five: Exercise

*This book is dedicated to all of you,
children and adults, who know what it is like
to live with diabetes on a daily basis,
and to those of you who are just learning.*

Acknowledgments

The authors would like to thank their many friends in the medical community for reviewing this book for accuracy and for their helpful suggestions. Special thanks go to Dr. Randy Dorian, Chief Science Officer at Hanuman Medical LLC, for his encouragement and tireless collaboration. Finally, we want to thank our editor, Carol A. Rosenberg, for her outstanding work.

How to Use This Book

This book is divided into several parts. As you progress from one part to the next, the complexity and the amount of information increases. Learn the basics in the first few parts and use the more technical parts as reference guides.

Part One is a simple overview of the principles you need to be aware of in caring for yourself. While it's geared for young people, everyone should read this part. It discusses many important aspects of living with diabetes. Part Two is a guide to nutrition and meal planning. It includes some tasty, "good-for-you" recipes. Part Three discusses diabetes a little more in depth and explains the different types of insulin and other medications used to control diabetes. Taking that one step further, it discusses various nutritional supplements that may help improve the condition. Part Four discusses the glycemic index and will help you to determine how different foods will affect your blood sugar levels. Part Five explains two types of exercise that have been shown to help people with diabetes: aerobic walking and weight-resistance training. Following Part Five is a section called "Terms to Know." This section recaps some of the definitions found in the book, but also includes some additional terms. Be sure to read this section. Finally, the book closes with a suggested reading list for those who are interested in learning more, and an index, which will help you turn to the pages that focus on what you want to know. Enjoy!

Introduction

Molly is a fourteen-year-old spot-nosed monkey who has had insulin-dependent diabetes for six years. She is fed a careful diet, receives insulin injections, and has her blood and urine tested regularly. All of these things were hard adjustments for her, just as they are for people with diabetes. Molly has a brittle (unstable) form of diabetes and is also insulin resistant. In spite of this, she has an upbeat, charming personality. Her gentleness and spirit of cooperation are priceless.

Your health, as well as the health of your loved ones, is of utmost importance. One purpose of this book is to let people with diabetes know that they are not alone. Another is to help inspire them to do the simple things they can do for their own care, including eating a proper diet that helps keep their blood sugar levels even.

All the factual information in this book has been drawn from scientific literature. Treat this book as an educational tool that will enable you to better understand and treat diabetes.

PART ONE

Understanding Diabetes

Molly's Story: How I Found Out I Have Diabetes

My name is Molly, and I'm a lot like you. I have diabetes, too.

At first I was thirsty and drank a lot of water! I was always hungry for something sweet!

My doctor ran a lot of tests. He said I had diabetes. So I needed to have my toe or finger pricked for blood tests to measure my blood sugar levels.

I followed my diet and exercise program, but it wasn't enough.

So I needed to take insulin, too.

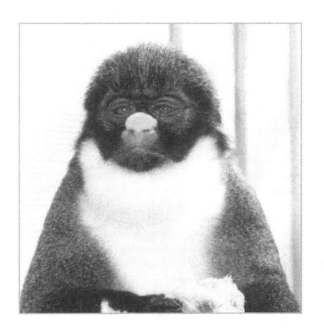

- Insulin is needed to convert sugar from food into the energy that runs our bodies.

- Type 1 diabetes means that your body cannot make insulin.

- Type 2 diabetes means that your body cannot properly use insulin.

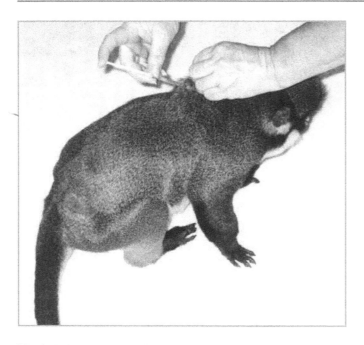

At first, I was afraid to take my insulin shots. I didn't understand why I had to have them. But now I'm not afraid.

I know I feel better with insulin. I need insulin to help my body use sugar, and I'm lucky to get it. Without insulin shots, I'd get very sick again.

Insulin is a hormone (or chemical messenger) made by a gland in the body called the *pancreas*. After you eat a meal or snack, insulin has some work to do. It regulates your blood sugar (glucose) by allowing it to leave the bloodstream and go into your cells, which use it as a source of energy.

Blood sugar, also called glucose, is needed by your cells for energy and proper function. It comes mainly from eating carbohydrates (like cereals and potatoes) or simple sugars (found in foods like fruit, honey, and table sugar). Some blood sugar also comes from eating proteins like meat and fish. (About half of the protein you eat can be converted to blood sugar.) A little blood sugar comes from fats like oil and butter. (About 10 percent of the fat you eat can be converted to blood sugar.)

Symptoms of Diabetes

TYPE 1 SYMPTOMS

When people first get sick from type 1 diabetes, they become unusually thirsty, urinate more often, become very hungry, lose weight, get tired more easily, and become irritable (or grouchy).

TYPE 2 SYMPTOMS

When people first get sick from type 2 diabetes, they often have no symptoms at all. This is because type 2 diabetes can develop gradually over a long period of time. As type 2 diabetes develops, vision (eyesight) may become blurry

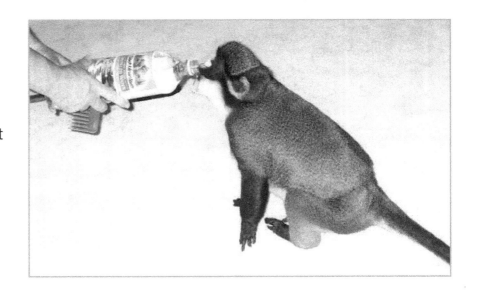

and cuts and bruises may be slow to heal. Some people may feel tingling or loss of feeling in their hands and feet. They may also have recurring skin, gum, or bladder infections. When their blood sugar levels are consistently too high, some people with type 2 diabetes also experience type 1 symptoms.

Insulin and the Pancreas

The pancreas is a gland that sits just behind the stomach. It has two main jobs. The first is to make substances called *enzymes*, which help in the digestion of food. The second job is to make insulin.

The pancreas is the only organ in the body that makes insulin. If it works properly, the pancreas makes just the right amount of insulin. The food we eat is digested by the body and turned into glucose (blood sugar). Insulin is needed to help get blood sugar into our cells for energy. If the amount of sugar in our bloodstream runs too high or too low, typically we feel bad (sometimes very sick), and our bodies do not function as well.

Sometimes I wish I had a normal pancreas....

Too much insulin causes blood sugar levels to drop (low blood sugar) and too little insulin causes blood sugar levels to go up (high blood sugar).

But the good news is . . . diabetes is treatable! Not all health problems can be treated, you know!

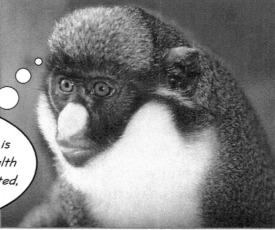

How Diabetes Is Treated

ORAL MEDICATIONS FOR TYPE 2 DIABETES ONLY

Many different oral medications are used to treat and manage different symptoms of type 2 diabetes. More than one oral medication may be taken, and the medications may be taken in combination with insulin.

INSULIN SHOTS FOR TYPE 1 OR TYPE 2 DIABETES

People with type 1 diabetes and some people with type 2 diabetes need to have insulin shots to help keep their blood sugar levels normal.

- All people with type 1 diabetes must use insulin.

- Some people with type 2 diabetes can control their diabetes with diet and exercise alone. But most use oral medicines, insulin, or both.

- People like me who take insulin need to have shots every day.

- Sometimes I need several shots a day. I get shots with superfine needles.

- I use two kinds of insulin, regular and mixed (70–30). There are now more than twenty kinds of insulin that your doctor will help you to choose from.

9

- Remember to wipe your skin with alcohol before you get a shot and to shake the bottle of insulin before filling the syringe!

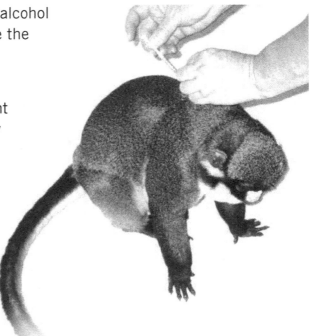

- I can take insulin shots in different places on my body. My back is my favorite spot. For people, the stomach is usually the best spot for insulin absorption.

- People with diabetes need to develop their own personal plan for diabetes treatment. Your doctor or healthcare team will help.

Safe Needle Disposal

Don't leave your used needles lying around where people might accidentally get poked. Here are two good ideas for getting rid of them safely:

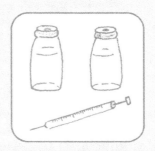

- ■ Wash out an empty laundry detergent bottle. They make great storage containers for used lancets and syringes.

- ■ Wash out an empty peanut butter jar or other similar-sized plastic jar. They make good disposal containers when traveling.

Monitoring Blood Sugar Levels

Scientists have shown that people with type 1 or type 2 diabetes can slow down (or keep from getting) many of the long-term health problems associated with diabetes just by keeping their blood sugar (glucose) levels normal.

Your doctor will tell you that blood sugar levels are considered within the normal range when they measure between 80 and 120 mg/dl after fasting (no food all night).

Remember, the goal is to keep blood sugar levels as close to normal as possible. Many things can cause changes in your blood sugar levels, including delayed meals, overeating, exercise, stress, sickness, lack of sleep, and changes in your diabetes medications.

BLOOD SUGAR MONITORS

You can buy a home glucose-testing product (like the one shown here) to help you test your blood sugar levels.

- Blood sugar monitors help you do the finger-stick test (explained on page 12).

- Try to buy a blood sugar monitor that is made to work with a small amount of blood.

- Some monitors even work with your computer to help you keep a record of your blood sugar levels!

- Some monitors display large numbers to make them easy to read.

- Choose a monitor that fits your needs and lifestyle best, and use it often to help you maintain normal blood sugar levels.

The Finger-Stick Test

To use your blood glucose monitor, you'll prick your finger and apply a drop of blood to the end of the strip. Your monitor will give you a number, which indicates how much sugar is in your blood. This do-it-yourself test is excellent because it measures your blood sugar at the time you test it. Your goal should be to keep your blood sugar levels as close to normal as possible.

When should I do the finger-stick test?

These are the best times to test:

- Before meals
- Before bed
- One to two hours after meals
- At 2 A.M. or 3 A.M. at least once a week if you have type 1 diabetes.

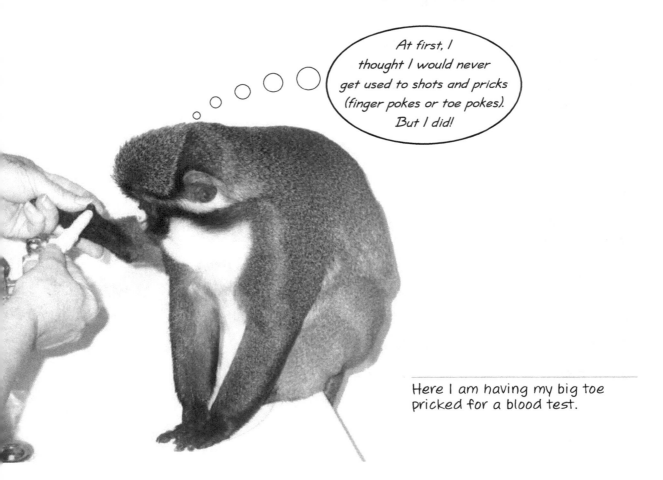

At first, I thought I would never get used to shots and pricks (finger pokes or toe pokes). But I did!

Here I am having my big toe pricked for a blood test.

Frequent Testing Is Best!

You may need extra tests before you exercise, when you suspect you have high or low blood sugar, if you wake up with high or low blood sugar levels, or when you're sick. The more often you test your blood sugar levels and make needed adjustments to your treatment program, the less likely you are to develop diabetes-associated health problems.

Monitoring with Test Strips

Urine Test Strips

Urine test strips can be used to test for sugars or *ketones.* When the test strip is dipped into urine, the test area changes color according to the amount of sugar or ketones in the urine. Using urine test strips for ketones is more common than using them to test for sugar levels. This is because urine sugar test strips have drawbacks:

1. Urine testing gives you some information on your sugar levels, but it is not as accurate or meaningful as blood testing.

2. Urine testing won't tell you if you have low blood sugar, but blood tests will.

3. Urine sugar readings change when your volume of urine changes (when you drink more fluids). This is one reason that they are not as accurate as blood tests.

4. Urine glucose levels are an average value of excess sugar that has spilled into your urine over the last few hours, whereas blood glucose testing gives the level of your blood sugar at that moment.

5. Sugar appears in your urine only when your blood sugar levels are very high.

Keto Strips

Keto strips give you a fast, easy way to test urine for ketones (something you don't want to find). Finding ketones will alert you to changes in your diabetes. You can use this information to make adjustments in your diet and medications to get rid of the ketones.

What Are Ketones?

Ketones (or ketone bodies) are acidic waste products produced when fatty acids are broken down for energy.

Ketones are one of the body's warnings that you need better diabetes management.

In someone with diabetes, the development of ketones can lead to a condition called *diabetic ketoacidosis.*

Diabetic Ketoacidosis

Diabetic ketoacidosis occurs when you don't have enough insulin to use glucose as a fuel to run your body. Body fat is used instead. The byproduct of using body fat as fuel is ketones. Ketones build up in the blood and spill over into the urine. Diabetic ketoacidosis develops when the blood is more acidic than the body tissues.

Diabetic ketoacidosis can be a life-threatening emergency. See your doctor immediately if you test positive for ketones and have any of these symptoms: increased thirst and urination, nausea, deep and rapid breathing, abdominal pain, sweet smelling breath, or loss of consciousness.

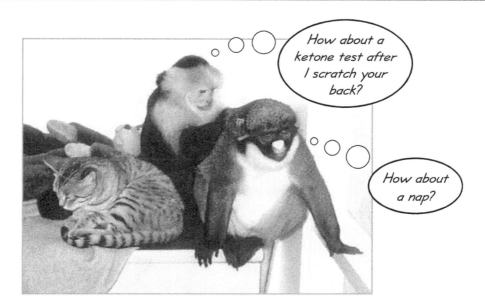

REMEMBER . . .

Healthcare professionals recommend blood glucose monitor tests over urine sugar tests. They show what your blood sugar is at that moment. Urine tests show how much excess sugar spilled into your urine over the last several hours.

You can use keto strips to test your ketone levels. People with type 1 diabetes need to test for ketones when they are experiencing symptoms, or if their blood sugar levels stay very high. **If your strip shows ketones, call your doctor!**

Type 1 (and Type 2) High and Low Blood Sugar Symptoms

(When blood sugar levels are consistently too high, some people with type 2 diabetes experience these type 1 symptoms.)

WARNING SIGNS THAT ARE EASY TO SEE

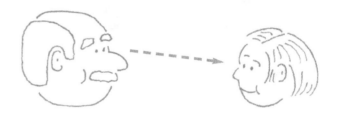

If you have low blood sugar, your skin might be pale, moist, or sweaty, and you may feel excited, shaky, grouchy, or confused. Your breathing could be anywhere from normal to rapid, and your breath odor will be normal.

If you have high blood sugar, your skin might be flushed and dry, and you may feel drowsy and tired. Your breathing could be deep, labored, or shallow. Your breath may have a fruity odor and you might vomit.

WARNING SIGNS THAT NEED A CLOSER LOOK

If you have low blood sugar, your tongue might be unusually moist, tingling, or numb, and you might be hungry. You also might have a headache.

If you have high blood sugar, your tongue will be dry, and you will be very thirsty. You will also need to urinate a lot. You might have a stomachache.

There are other signs that you have had either too much or not enough insulin. Signs can vary in different people.

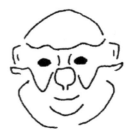

- When I have low blood sugar, I act tired or confused.

- When my blood sugar is a bit high, I want to eat sweet foods or I eat too much. When it's dangerously high, I am not hungry.

WHEN I HAVE HIGH BLOOD SUGAR . . .

If I am experiencing symptoms of high blood sugar, I take a blood test. Then, I take an extra insulin injection. The amount of insulin I need depends on how high my blood sugar levels are. I have to be careful since too much insulin will cause low blood sugar.

WHEN I HAVE LOW BLOOD SUGAR . . .

If our insulin levels get too high (if we take too much insulin or too much diabetes medication), we may feel tired, shaky, or hungry due to low blood sugar. If this happens to me, I need to pop a glucose tab right away. (Glucose tabs are commercially measured out sugar tablets available at drugstores.) Many diabetes healthcare professionals recommend glucose tabs, because they work quickly and come in a premeasured dose. Some foods will also bring your blood sugar levels back up (see page 18).

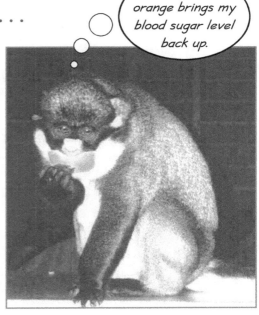

A slice of orange brings my blood sugar level back up.

BRINGING BLOOD SUGAR LEVELS BACK UP

Foods to eat *only* when your blood sugar is dangerously low:

- ❏ Three or four glucose tabs
- ❏ A small box of raisins
- ❏ A wedge of sweet fruit or a fruit roll-up
- ❏ Four or five dates
- ❏ Plain yogurt, non-fat or low-fat, with mashed berries and a few nuts

Foods to eat when your blood sugar goes just a little bit too low:

- ❏ Cheese or peanut butter with whole-grain crackers
- ❏ Nuts mixed with fresh fruit (like peanuts and a fruit wedge)
- ❏ Puffed rice cakes, plain or flavored

Eating Smart

People with diabetes need to be smarter than most people about the foods they eat. We need to know which foods belong to which food groups so that we can eat smart! You can learn some of what you need to know right here, but there's even more information about eating right in Part Two.

Anyone who has diabetes can benefit by following a smart eating plan. (Eating smart is better for everyone, even for people without diabetes!) Many people with type 2 diabetes will be able to take less medication or even stop taking it (with their doctors' permission, of course) if they follow a smart eating plan.

FOOD GROUPS FOR PEOPLE WITH DIABETES

1. Proteins
2. Dairy
3. Low-Carb Veggies
4. High-Carb Veggies and Legumes
5. Complex Carbs (Grains)
6. Fruit
7. Fat
8. Fiber
9. Free Food

First learn your food groups. Then learn to balance them!

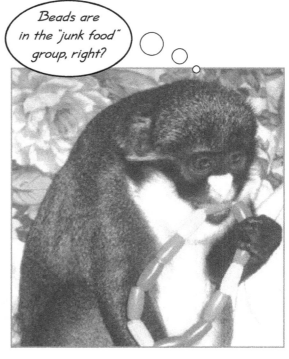

EATING SMART MEANS . . .

The food you eat can help keep your blood sugar levels more even. It's easy!

- Keep blood sugar levels even by balancing your food groups at each meal or snack. Be sure to include fiber *and* protein in every meal and snack you eat! Fiber is built into whole grains and legumes. It's also in veggies and whole fruits (not fruit juices)—especially when you eat them raw!

- Try not to eat refined sugar and flour products, better known as "junk food." Instead, eat healthful carbohydrates (or "carbs" for short).

- Don't eat too much fat, and be careful about the kind of fat you eat. There are "good" fats and "bad" fats.

- Try not to overeat! Enjoy your foods and eat just the right amount for your body.

A Good Idea!

People with diabetes need a smart food plan so they can eat the right foods at the right times. You can use your imagination to plan your meals. Just for fun, start your new food plan with the following craft project. This is a good way to get everyone in your family involved.

FOOD-PLANNING CRAFT PROJECT

1. Using a nontoxic felt pen, divide a paper plate into three sections like a pie, and draw a circle in the center.

2. For a breakfast plate, label the three sections "Protein," "Carbs," and "Dairy." Label the circle in the center "Fat." For a dinner or lunch plate, label the three sections "Protein," "Carbs," and "Veggies." Again, label the circle in the center "Fat."

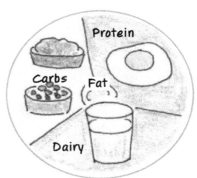

BREAKFAST

3. Choose the foods that you like from Molly's lists in Part Two. You can either draw these foods in the proper sections of the plate or simply write them in. Then, color in your plates. Plates can be used for serving or you can place a clear plastic plate over your paper plate.

4. Keep the finished plates in a large plastic bag and save them for meal and snack ideas. At meal time, try to copy your craft project ideas onto your real plate.

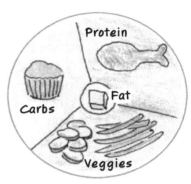

LUNCH or DINNER

Food-Planning Ideas

- In the protein section, put fish, lean meat, sugar-free protein powders, low-carb protein bars, whole eggs, and egg whites. Vegetarians (people who don't eat meat) may use tofu and milk products as protein sources. These have some carbs as well as protein.

- In the carb section, put whole grains and legumes. Some legumes are kidney beans, navy beans, garbanzo beans, lentils, garden peas, and split peas. This section is also for fruits and high-carb veggies like potatoes, yams, corn, and peas.

It's a Fact

An excellent way to keep your blood sugar level more even is to eat your protein first and your carbs second. If you want, your fat and low-carb veggies can be eaten at the same time you eat your protein.

- In the veggie section, put low-carb veggies, such as salad greens, celery, cucumber, bell peppers, broccoli, cauliflower, and green beans.

- In the fat section, put "good" fats such as Earth's Best margarine (or another brand of non-hydrogenated margarine). Olive oil, canola oil, and nut butter are also good fats.

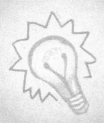

A Good Idea!
EATING BALANCED MEALS

❋ FOCUS! If following a balanced meal plan is new to you, have a positive attitude. Tell yourself, "I will just try this one day at a time starting today."

❋ At first, some people are likely to miss the excess carbs and junk foods, and you might be one of them. Do it "one meal at a time." Stick it out! You're worth it!

❋ Try to eat balanced meals for thirty days. You will notice a difference in your blood sugar level and in the way you feel.

❋ Have an "attitude of gratitude." With diabetes, your health is always improved with good diet. What a simple thing! Everyone who has a health problem should be so lucky!

> If I focus, I can balance my food groups just for today.

A Quick Review

To help keep your blood sugar levels even, eat low-fat foods, balance your protein with your carbs, and always include fiber in every meal and snack!

Smart Snacking

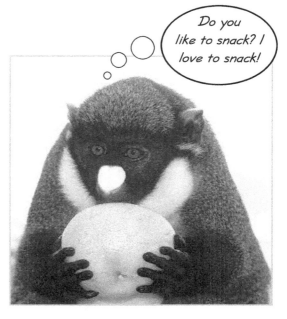

Do you like to snack? I love to snack!

I sometimes snack on "free foods," which are mainly low-carb veggies like celery and cucumber wedges.

THE BEST SNACKS ARE BALANCED SNACKS

Remember, a balanced snack includes a protein, a high-fiber carb, a little good fat, and maybe a fruit or veggie.

GREAT SNACKS

Try celery with peanut butter, or try whole-grain crackers with low-fat cheese or low-fat deli meat. Fill a whole-grain pita pocket with low-fat deli meat and salad or fill it with egg salad and shredded lettuce. Try strawberries on top of low-fat cottage cheese. Also, be sure to try some of my recipes!

When you snack on regular foods, you may need to take extra diabetes medication or an extra insulin shot.

FREE FOODS (TO GO WITH SNACKS OR MEALS)

- Cinnamon and mint tea
- Sugar-free sodas and teas
- Sugar-free Jell-O (up to 1 cup a day)
- Salsa for dipping veggies
- Dill pickles

⚖️ Balance Your Snack Attacks!

For tasty, balanced whole-grain cracker snacks, place a bed of curly lettuce on a cracker and top with a mixture of cottage cheese and fruit.

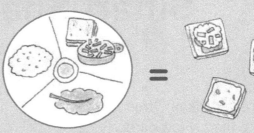

Snack on a funny-faced sandwich: Spread mayo on a piece of whole-grain bread. Lay a cooked hamburger patty on top. Use lettuce for the hair, a tomato for the mouth, olives for the eyes, and a pickle for the nose. . . . Yum!

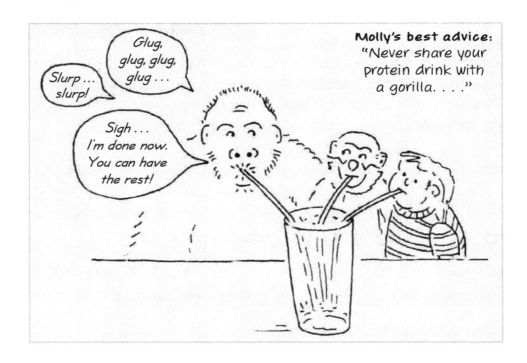

SIMPLE SNACK RECIPES

Here are some simple recipes you can try. You'll find even more recipes in Part Two!

MOLLY'S FAVORITE PROTEIN-BALANCED COTTAGE CHEESE & FRUIT

Makes 1 serving.

½ cup frozen strawberries or blueberries
or ½ cup canned (sugar-free) pineapple chunks

1 packet artificial sweetener, such as Splenda

½ cup low-fat cottage cheese*

Guar gum (optional)

*Organic cottage cheese is my favorite kind!

Thaw the berries just slightly in a microwave oven (about 20 seconds on high). Mash with a fork. (Don't microwave the pineapple chunks; just mash them.) Mix in the sweetener. Pour sweetened fruit over a scoop of cottage cheese. Sprinkle a bit of guar gum over the top for fiber, if desired. *It's delicious!*

PROTEIN-BALANCED YOGURT & FRUIT

Makes 1 serving.

½ cup frozen strawberries or blueberries

2 packets artificial sweetener, such as Splenda

½ cup low-fat plain yogurt*

1–2 tablespoons chopped walnuts

Flaxseed meal (optional)

*Organic yogurt is the healthiest kind.

Thaw the berries just slightly in a microwave oven (about 20 seconds on high). Mash with a fork. Mix in the sweetener. Stir in the yogurt. Sprinkle walnuts and a bit of flaxseed meal over the top for fiber, if desired. *It's great!*

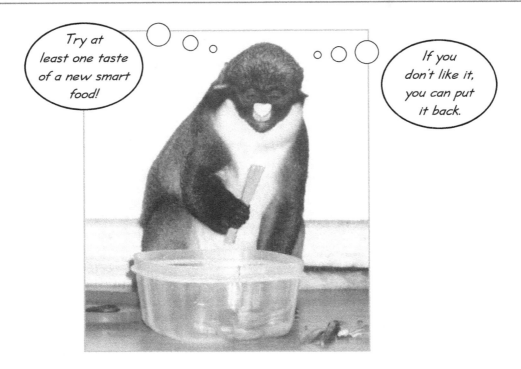

WHEN IT'S HARD TO EAT SMART . . .

It was hard for me to make the change from my favorite foods to smart foods. This is what I do when "smart" foods are not my favorite foods:

❀ I take a "test bite." Then I can say "no thanks" if I don't like it.

❀ I like to have many smart food choices. If I have at least two food choices, I eat the one I like best.

❀ I ask for lots of praise from others for eating new smart foods!

❀ I watch for smart food choices in those who eat with me. Good examples make it easier for me to eat smart! "Monkey see, monkey do!"

❀ I eat small meals and small snacks. I love finger foods like veggie, cheese, or meat strips!

❀ Sometimes I have my veggies first and my favorite smart foods second!

My "Try-Not-to-Eat" List

People with diabetes need a "try-not-to-eat" list—a list of foods that they should avoid. My "try-not-to-eat" list has a lot of concentrated sugary foods that make my blood sugar levels go up more easily than "good-for-you" balanced meals and snacks. Your list doesn't have to be exactly like mine, but you can use it as a guide.

MY "TRY-NOT-TO-EAT" LIST

- ✗ Candy
- ✗ Cookies and pastries
- ✗ Doughnuts
- ✗ Fatty fried foods
- ✗ Honey
- ✗ Jam and jelly
- ✗ Molasses
- ✗ Most dried fruit
- ✗ Puddings, pies, cakes
- ✗ Sugar
- ✗ Sugar-sweetened chewing gum
- ✗ Sugar-sweetened soft drinks
- ✗ Sugar-coated cereals
- ✗ Syrups
- ✗ White flour breads

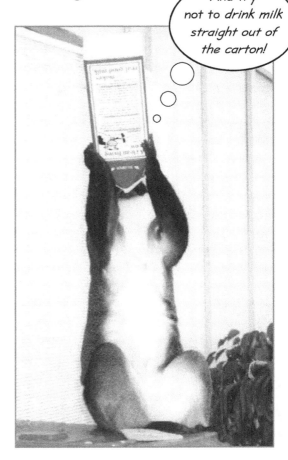

And try not to drink milk straight out of the carton!

Your "Try-Not-to-Eat" List

X

X

X

X

X

X

X

X

X

X

X

X

X

X

X

X

X

X

X

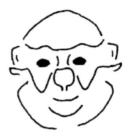

It's a Fact

If you're like me, at first you might like mainly the foods on your "Try-Not-to-Eat" list. But if you leave the junk food out of your diet, your taste buds will change! You will start to like, or even love, the taste of "real food" like meat, fruits, veggies, and whole grains!

My Exercise Plan

People with diabetes need daily exercise. (For more information, see Part Five: Exercise.) It helps the blood to circulate and helps insulin to work its best. People with diabetes need an exercise plan. What's yours?

⚽ My serious exercise plan includes running, jumping, climbing trees, playing in the sand, adventure walking, swimming, and chasing other monkeys.

⚽ My not-so-serious exercise plan includes sitting (is sitting an exercise?) and eating (really!).

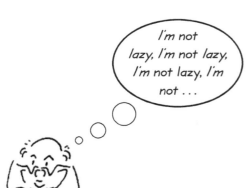

I'm not lazy, I'm not lazy, I'm not lazy, I'm not . . .

REMEMBER:

If you run, swim, ride your bike, play tennis, play field sports, do aerobics, or engage in other exercise, your body will use your insulin better!

JUST SAY *YES* TO EXERCISE!

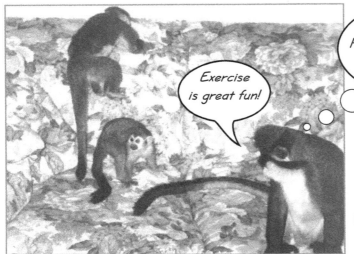

Exercise is great fun!

I could play leap frog, go dancing, or do kung fu.

I could go exploring . . . play basketball, swim, or jog.

When all else fails, a simple walk will do!

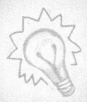

A Good Idea!

Make yourself a daily exercise chart. (See the chart on the next page.) Fill in the first column with some of the exercise ideas below:

☀ aerobic walking	☀ aerobics	☀ baseball	☀ basketball
☀ belly dancing	☀ biking	☀ bowling	☀ boxing
☀ dancing	☀ downhill skiing	☀ fencing	☀ football
☀ golf	☀ gymnastics	☀ karate	☀ kick boxing
☀ kung fu	☀ rowing	☀ running	☀ skateboarding
☀ skating	☀ soccer	☀ softball	☀ surfing
☀ swimming	☀ tennis	☀ track and field	☀ volleyball
☀ weight lifting	☀ wrestling		

YOUR EXERCISE CHART

Here's an exercise chart you can use any time! Fill in the types of exercises you like to do in the first column. Then, copy the chart on a copy machine so you have extras! Draw or paste a star in the proper row every time you do an exercise on a particular day. When you get ten stars, ask a friend or someone in your family to take you out for a special outing or activity!

Guess which sport is one of the best sports for a total body workout...

BASKETBALL!

Exercise	Mon	Tue	Wed	Thu	Fri	Sat	Sun

I'll rest up first, then I'll go for a little jog...

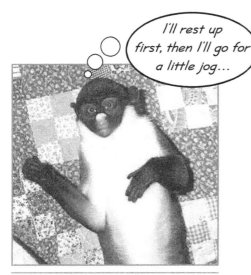

This is me when I was little.

A Good Idea!

EXERCISE: YOU CAN DO IT!

☀ Exercise at the time of day when you have the most energy.

☀ Rest up for exercise if you need to!

☀ Set aside a time slot for each exercise. A half hour is enough!

☀ Say to yourself, "Just for today, I can do this!"

☀ Make it fun! Exercise to music!

The Importance of Grooming

- It's extra important for people with diabetes to take good care of their skin and teeth. I like to keep my skin clean . . . and I like to get my fur combed.

- Be sure to take extra care of any sores you might have. Have your doctor check all of your sores and wounds.

- Remember to brush and floss your teeth. Ask your dentist to show you how to floss. Use a soft toothbrush. Hard ones can scratch your gums!

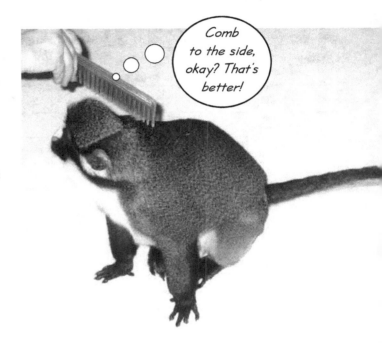

- Cigarette smoke is very bad for our hearts and circulation. Stay away from secondhand smoke! This is very important! If someone you know smokes, he or she should smoke outside, not inside your house.

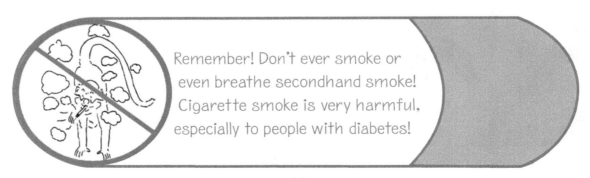

Remember! Don't ever smoke or even breathe secondhand smoke! Cigarette smoke is very harmful, especially to people with diabetes!

My Friends and My Diabetes

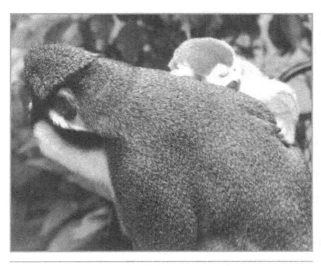

This is my friend Pip.

Do your friends know about your diabetes? My friend Heidi thinks insulin shots are special, so she likes to get pretend shots.

All of your friends should know you have diabetes.

- Between shots and toe pricks, I do many regular things, like swinging around my jungle gym, playing with electronic toys, and hanging out with my friends.

- In case my blood sugar level ever gets dangerously high, everyone I know (teachers, caregivers, close neighbors, and friends) knows that I need insulin. And when my blood sugar gets low, they know I need to take a glucose tab or eat a snack.

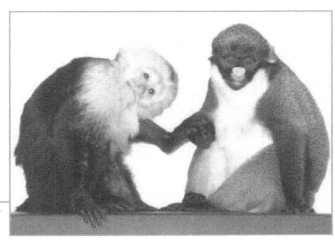

In this picture, Heidi gave me her foot to hold instead of her hand.

Telling Friends . . .

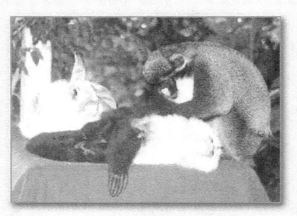

Sharing information about diabetes with your friends is a good way to get closer to people you care about who care about you!

You might start by asking your friend, "Have you ever had a health problem that you needed to take medicine for or that you had to see a doctor for?" (Most of your friends probably have.)

Ask if it was something someone could catch, like a cold. Find out how long your friend had this health problem and what he or she did to take care of it.

Then you can tell your friend that you have a health problem and that it's not something your friend can catch from you. Ask your friend if he or she has ever heard of diabetes. Then say, "Diabetes is a health problem that doesn't go away, but it's one where you can be healthy if you take good care of yourself and follow your doctor's advice!" You can even show this book to your friend!

Diabetes Gear

Gear bags help with better diabetes management. An effective gear bag contains everything you might need for your personal on-the-spot diabetes care.

Put everything you need in your gear bag, but don't put in anything extra. You want to be able to find important gear quickly and easily without going through extra items!

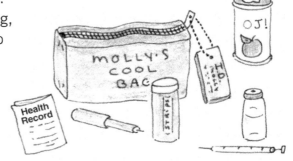

Take your gear bag with you wherever you go so that your insulin or medication will always be on hand if you start to have any diabetes-related symptoms.

A handy gear bag means you can take care of your blood sugar levels right away before you feel worse. If you had to wait till you got home for your gear, you would take the risk of increasingly worse symptoms.

In case you need help someday, explain how to use your special gear to family members, teachers, close neighbors, and friends.

Put everything you need in your gear bag, but don't put in anything extra! (No toys and no old socks, okay?)

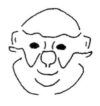

A Good Idea!

Have some fun! Get an extra cool kit or bag for your diabetes gear. Use adhesive stars or other bright stickers to color code the gear you will need for emergencies.

Keeping Insulin in Gear Bags

When going out, choose the best way for you to take your gear bag along. A backpack, a waist pouch, a carrying case, a big pocket, or a purse will work.

Insulin must be carried and stored with care. All types of insulin can be ruined by excessive heat or freezing temperatures. Never leave insulin in the glove compartment in a car; temperature extremes can cause the insulin to spoil. For cold weather travel, keep your insulin in a pocket close to your body. In really hot weather, carry a cooler with an icepack; be sure the insulin is kept cool but does not freeze.

GEAR CHECKLIST FOR TRIPS AND SLEEPOVERS

❏ Your identification tag

❏ Insulin (including an extra bottle in case of breakage) and syringes

❏ Alcohol wipes

❏ Finger-pricking device and meter

❏ Urine test strips

❏ Any medications or prescriptions

❏ Some glucose tabs in case of too much insulin

❏ A copy of your health record and doctor's phone number

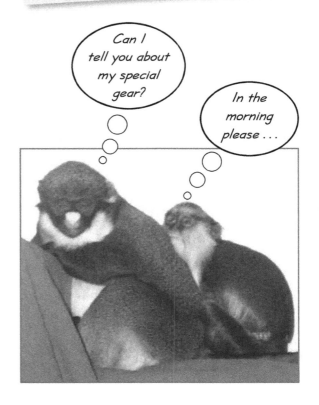

Can I tell you about my special gear?

In the morning please . . .

My Feelings

Expressing a wide range of feelings is part of being a healthy and mature person. But did you know that STRONG feelings like being mad, scared, or excited can make your blood sugar levels go up? Sometimes, they can make your blood sugar levels fall. Here is a list of some feelings that can change your blood sugar levels:

- Anger
- Disappointment
- Excitement

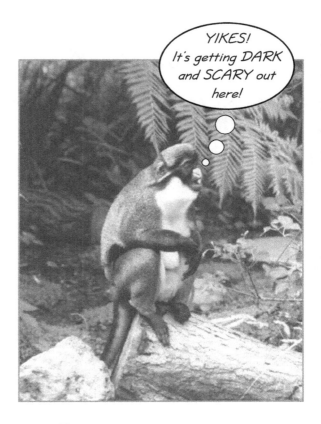

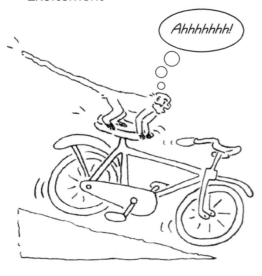

- Fear
- Jealousy
- Joy
- Sadness
- A lot of strong feelings all at once

Things to Do and Remember

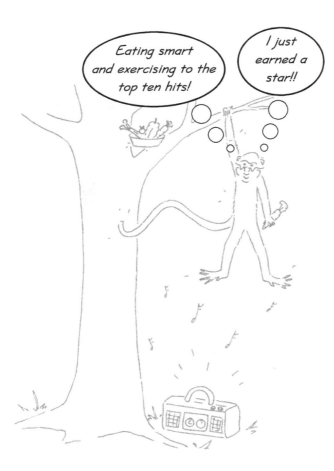

⭐ Getting shots and pricks is not one of my favorite things, but I'm used to them now. I also know how important they are.

⭐ No matter how old you are, remind your family to give you lots of praise (and sometimes pats and hugs) when you follow a diabetes procedure. Make sure you get praise for improvement! It really helps!

⭐ No matter how old you are, make yourself a star chart! (See below.) Even grown-ups like star charts! They help remind you what a good job you are doing with your care! Every time you do something difficult, think to yourself, "I just earned a star!"

MAKE A STAR CHART!

Draw out your chart on any kind of paper (poster board works well) or photocopy the chart on page 39. Use refrigerator magnets to attach your star chart to the fridge. Buy adhesive stars or other colorful stickers. Paste one into the chart every time you do something to care for yourself.

	Mon	Tue	Wed	Thu	Fri	Sat	Sun
Balanced my meals							
Balanced my snacks							
Exercised							
Took my blood tests							
Took my insulin (or diabetes meds) on time							
Had my gear bag when I went out							
Had an upbeat attitude							

I GOT ATTITUDE!

To have an upbeat attitude . . . exercise it! It's like a muscle that gets stronger when you do! If you start to feel down, take a minute and think of a few positive things in a row! Your list might go like this: "I am happy to have my friend Jo (or anything positive about a friend or relative). I enjoyed the beautiful trees and sky I saw today (or anything from nature). I am grateful for my fingers (or anything about yourself) that bend and work perfectly."

Smile! . . . You just had an attitude adjustment!

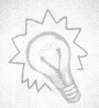

A Good Idea!

People like us with diabetes need to keep a record book. My record book shows my food plan. It shows my shots and pricks. And it shows how my blood sugar is doing. Have you started a record book? If not, now's a good time!

In addition to recording your blood sugar readings, you'll want to make a note of whether you felt sick, tired, or stressed; what kind of exercise you did and for how long; and whether you ate more or less than you usually do (all of the factors that are likely to affect your blood sugar).

MORE THINGS TO REMEMBER

1. I can learn to have an upbeat attitude, and so can you!

2. I can be smart and successful! The best prescription for success is to eat smart, exercise daily, and test your blood sugar levels often.

3. For the best care, ask someone to help you with the details of a smart food plan that includes foods you like.

4. Scientists are working hard to find a cure for people with diabetes! Meanwhile, the best advice is to take good care of yourself!

5. Diabetes doesn't have to take over your life. I have plenty of time for my friends, for fun, and for just hanging out!

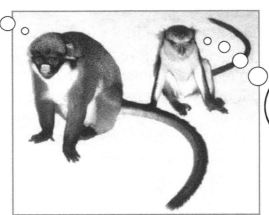

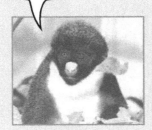

I Would Love to Hear from YOU!

♥ Please visit my website and e-mail me a letter about yourself. You can even send me a picture. You can also ask me any question you have about this book.

Your friend, Molly the Monkey

molly@hellomolly.com

PART TWO

Nutrition for Diabetes

An Introduction to Food Groups

People with diabetes need to learn about the different food groups. Even if nutrition is not a strong interest of yours, you can still learn how to eat properly! It's one of the keys to excellent management and care of diabetes.

Food Groups for People with Diabetes

1. Proteins
2. Dairy
3. Low-Carb Veggies
4. High-Carb Veggies and Legumes
5. Complex Carbs (Grains)
6. Fruit
7. Fat
8. Fiber (built into numbers 4, 5, and 6)
9. Free Food

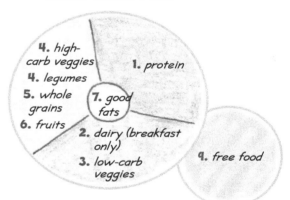

Basic Meal Plan

Make a Food Plan Every Day

Take fifteen minutes to plan your meals. A daily food plan is the best way to make sure that you always have balanced meals and snacks. Visualize your plate divided into four sections. You can have more than one type of carb if the amounts are small enough to fit in the carb section.

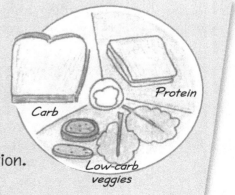

Food Planning

Plan your eats and eat your plan.

Diabetic Food Exchanges

Some people with diabetes use a diabetic food exchange list, and they learn to measure or weigh their food portions in order to have good blood sugar control. Food exchanges are a way to help people stay on special food plans by letting them replace one food from an exchange group with another from the same group. Look up food exchanges at www.hellomolly.com or get a list from your library or from your doctor.

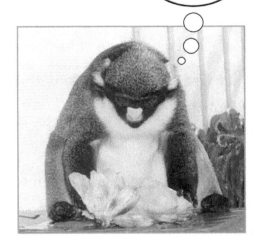

Glycemic Index

Some people with diabetes use the glycemic index. The glycemic index refers to the immediate rise in blood sugar that occurs as a result of eating a food high in carbohydrate. Foods that digest rapidly lead to a fast release of glucose into your bloodstream. These are known as high glycemic index foods. Foods that digest more slowly release glucose into your bloodstream gradually and are known as low glycemic index foods. (See page 99 for more on the glycemic index.)

A Good Idea!

MEASURE YOUR FOOD TO TRAIN YOUR EYE
Try measuring your food with a kitchen scale (or with measuring cups and spoons) for a few weeks. Measuring your food will help to train your eye to recognize food portions. After a while, you will no longer need to measure your food.

FOOD PLAN CHART

For added food-planning support, use a notebook to record your food plans. Keep track of your meals on paper until you get used to planning.

Use the sample food plan chart below as a guideline.

SAMPLE DAILY FOOD PLAN CHART					
Breakfast	**Snack**	**Lunch**	**Snack**	**Dinner**	**Snack**
one egg ½ cup slow-cooking oats 1 cup of milk	low-fat cottage cheese and berries	water-packed tuna on 1 slice whole-grain bread with raw veggies, flax, and olive oil dressing	nut butter and celery	skinless baked chicken ½ potato green salad olive oil dressing	whole-grain crackers and low-fat cheese

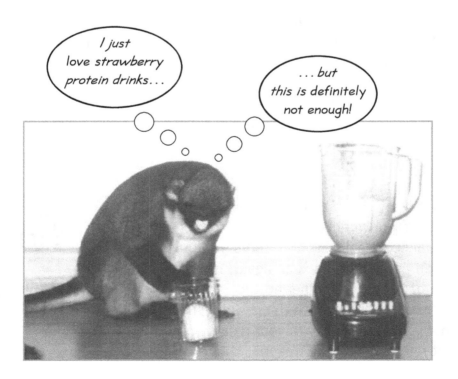

A Word about Calories and Overeating

Calories are the amount of available energy in food. Your doctor or nutritionist can work with you to find out roughly how many calories you use each day. You will want to work toward finding your ideal weight and staying there. Balancing the amount of food you eat with your physical activity will help you to maintain a proper body weight.

OVEREATING

The amount of food you eat is closely related to blood sugar control. If you overeat, your blood sugar goes up. Although carbs have the most effect on your blood sugar levels, the calories from overeating any type of food will cause your blood sugar level to go up!

Molly's best advice is to eat in moderation. Make a list of which foods tempt you to eat more. It's not spinach and broccoli, right? Help control your appetite by staying away from the greatest temptations: high-sugar foods, high-glycemic carbs, and high-fat foods (junk foods). They tend to make people want more! Keep doing the best you can to follow your balanced food plan and get regular, fun exercise!

DO I HAVE TO BE PERFECT?

No! There's an old saying: "Strive for progress—not perfection!" So it's not whether or not you occasionally fall off the "balanced meal wagon" . . . it's how quickly you pick yourself up and get back on again! If your eating gets out of hand, try another attitude adjustment. Make a list of three positive things you can say to yourself that you have done with your meals in the past! Then get right back on the wagon!

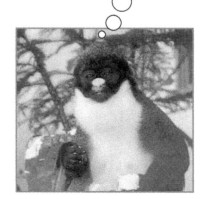

Oops, I'm not perfect.

Molly's Popular Protein Foods

Most proteins, even lean ones, also have a small amount of fat. Always buy lean cuts of meat and trim any visible fat. These all-protein foods have no fiber, so eat them with a high-fiber carb or veggie:

- Lean chicken
- Lean turkey
- Lean beef
- Lean pork
- Lean hot dogs
- Fish
- Tofu (has some carbs too)

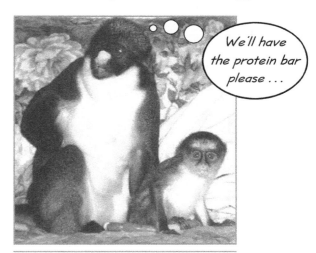

We'll have the protein bar please ...

This is me with Sasha when she was just a baby.

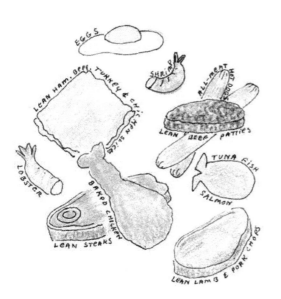

- Eggs, especially egg whites and egg substitute (see Molly's Smart Dairy Foods on page 48)

- Low-carb protein bars (see Food Products Molly Recommends on page 74)

- Sugar-free protein powders (see Food Products Molly Recommends on page 74)

47

Molly's Smart Dairy Foods

- Low-fat milk*

- Lactaid milk*

- Low-fat yogurt*

- Low-fat cottage cheese

- Low-fat cheese and cream cheese

- Low-fat or fat-free sour cream

- Low-fat ricotta cheese

- All-whey protein powder (comes in vanilla, chocolate, and berry flavors)

*high enough in carbs to make your blood sugar levels go up, so consider mixing a spoonful of low-carb protein powder into dairy foods to give them a higher protein-to-carbohydrate ratio.

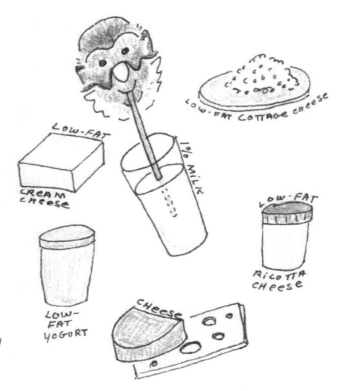

✔ Keep in mind that in addition to protein, all dairy products have some carbs and most have some fat (unless they are fat-free). The best choices are 1% fat or fat-free dairy products.

✔ Milk and yogurt are high in carbohydrates and are used quickly by the body.

✔ Organic, hormone-free dairy products are the best for your health.

✔ Dairy products have no fiber, so have them with some high-fiber foods like whole-grain carbs, fruits, or veggies!

✔ If you are lactose intolerant, your body cannot tolerate the milk sugar found in dairy products. There are many natural products available that can help make eating dairy products less of a problem for you.

A Good Idea!

When using milk on cereal, consider adding 2 tablespoons of unsweetened vanilla whey protein powder. It's great tasting and adds protein to the milk to help keep your blood sugar levels even!

Molly's Low-Carb Veggies

- Arugula
- Asparagus
- Bamboo shoots
- Bean sprouts
- Bok choy
- Broccoli
- Brussels sprouts
- Cabbage
- Cauliflower
- Celery
- Chicory
- Cilantro
- Cucumber
- Eggplant
- Endive
- Escarole
- Green or wax beans
- Green pepper
- Greens (all)
- Head lettuce
- Jerusalem artichoke
- Jicama
- Kohlrabi
- Mushrooms
- Okra
- Parsley
- Pea pods
- Radishes
- Red pepper
- Rhubarb (no sugar)
- Romaine lettuce
- Scallions
- Spinach
- Summer squash
- Swiss chard
- Tomato (raw)
- Water cress
- Yellow pepper
- Zucchini squash

✔ The foods listed above contain very few carbs. They are also "slow-burning," or low-glycemic carbs, the best kind to help keep your blood sugar levels even.

✔ Find at least one or two low-carb veggies that you like.

✔ I like sliced cucumber, celery, and cooked green beans!

✔ Low-carb veggies also contain some fiber.

• Try celery with peanut butter or celery in a stir-fry with chicken.

• Eat spinach sautéed in sesame oil.

• Bell pepper is good stuffed with brown rice and cooked ground meat.

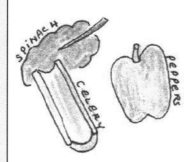

• Use tomatoes to make mild salsa and eat the salsa with Spanish beans and brown rice!

• Make a dip for raw veggies by mixing together roasted eggplant, yogurt, and mayonnaise!

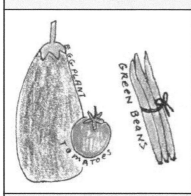

• Eat cabbage or cauliflower sautéed in a teaspoon of sesame oil.

• Eat broccoli sautéed in olive oil.

• Green beans are good sautéed in olive oil. Or steam them and spread them over a green salad.

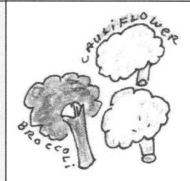

• Try cucumbers with my yogurt dressing. (See page 72.) You can dip raw celery and cauliflower in the dressing, too.

• Chop some parsley or cilantro to flavor your salsa! Or chop the herbs and sprinkle them on a baked potato.

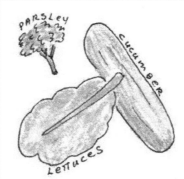

• Introduce all new salad vegetables by chopping them finely. Sprinkle just a tablespoon over cottage cheese and berries to see if you like the new vegetable.

Molly's High-Carb Veggies and Legumes

VEGETABLES

- Beets
- Pumpkin
- Cooked carrots
- Sweet potatoes
- Onions
- Turnips
- Peas
- Winter squashes
- Potatoes
- Yams

LEGUMES

- dried peas
- lentils
- kidney beans

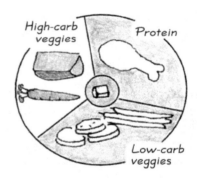

High-carb veggies / Protein / Low-carb veggies

✔ High-carb veggies (also called starchy veggies) are not free foods.

✔ High-carb veggies do have some fiber.

✔ In addition to having more carbs, high-carb veggies also have more calories than low-carb veggies.

✔ High-carb veggies are "fast energy" or "high glycemic" and should not be eaten on an empty stomach or without protein foods.

✔ They can make a nutritious part of a balanced meal if eaten in reasonable amounts.

✔ Legumes are high in carbs but are also high in fiber. You still need to balance them with protein and a good fat.

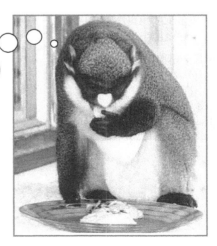

Mmmm... potato!

52

Molly's Favorite Complex Carbs

- ½ cup old-fashioned oatmeal
- Seven-grain bread (1 slice)
- ½ cup whole-grain pasta
- ⅓ cup brown rice
- ½ whole-grain pita pocket
- Complex carbs are more nutritious and have more fiber than refined or junk food carbs (made with white flour and sugar).

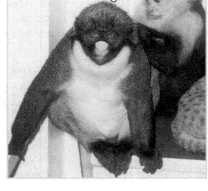

Pick a carb, any carb!

WHOLE GRAINS

Since whole grains (complex carbs) turn into glucose in the body more slowly than refined carbs, they are the best carbohydrate choices. But even though whole grains have more vitamins, minerals, and fiber, we still need to balance all our carbs with protein, good fats, and low-carb veggies!

How to Eat More Whole Grains

✔ Replace white rice with brown rice, millet pilaf, bulgur pilaf, or kasha.

✔ Replace saltine crackers with whole-grain wheat (like Ak-Mak) or rye crackers.

✔ Replace presweetened cereals with old-fashioned oatmeal or other whole-grain cereals.

✔ Replace white bread with seven- or nine-grain breads or other whole-grain breads.

✔ Replace cakes and pastries with oat bran muffins or high-fiber bagels. Eat these with some low-fat protein (low-fat meat, fish, or dairy) and you will have a balanced snack!

A Carbohydrate Review

Q: How much of the food we eat turns to sugar in our bodies?

A: Almost 100 percent of the carbohydrates in foods you eat is converted to sugar (glucose) in the body, while only about 50 percent of the protein you eat and 10 percent of the fat you eat may be converted into sugar. Here's a "Carbohydrate Equation" to help you remember.

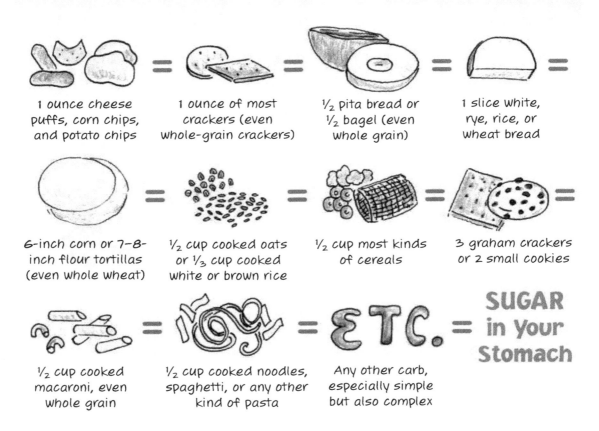

1 ounce cheese puffs, corn chips, and potato chips = 1 ounce of most crackers (even whole-grain crackers) = ½ pita bread or ½ bagel (even whole grain) = 1 slice white, rye, rice, or wheat bread =

6-inch corn or 7–8-inch flour tortillas (even whole wheat) = ½ cup cooked oats or ⅓ cup cooked white or brown rice = ½ cup most kinds of cereals = 3 graham crackers or 2 small cookies =

½ cup cooked macaroni, even whole grain = ½ cup cooked noodles, spaghetti, or any other kind of pasta = ETC. = Any other carb, especially simple but also complex = SUGAR in Your Stomach

In other words, the amount of sugar you eat is not the only thing that you have to watch. The body will convert all carbohydrates into glucose.

Molly's Smart Fruits

- Apples
- Oranges
- Blueberries
- Peaches
- Grapefruits
- Pears
- Grapes
- Strawberries

(all unsweetened)

✔ These fruits are low-sugar fruits. They are more "slow burning," or low glycemic, than sweet fruits (see below). They're the best kind for people with diabetes.

✔ Find at least one or two low-sugar fruits that you like!

✔ Practically all fruits are fat free and have some fiber.

✔ I love blueberries most of all!

I'd rather be eating blueberries . . .

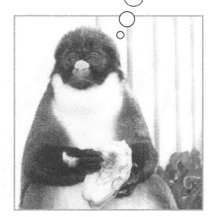

Sweet Fruits

- Banana
- Figs
- Mango
- Pineapple
- Cantaloupe
- Kiwi
- Papaya
- Watermelon

(all unsweetened)

- Sweet fruits are more "fast energy," or high glycemic. Eat them sparingly and, as with all fruits, as part of a balanced meal or snack.

  - All fruits have carbs but sweet fruits have the most.

Molly's Fat Facts in a Nutshell

Fat is a basic nutrient necessary for life. It has many important functions in the body, including helping in the absorption and transport of the fat-soluble vitamins A, D, E, and K through the bloodstream. Healthy skin and hair are maintained by fat. Your body uses fats to help build hormones and to build cell walls, and fat is an important source of energy.

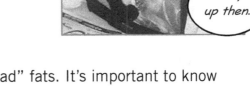

First we'll groom, then we'll have a "good fat" snack!

Hurry up then.

✔ People with diabetes know they should keep their diets low in fat. But people are also learning that the *kind* of fat you eat makes a difference.

✔ Some fats are "good" fats and some are "bad" fats. It's important to know which fats are "good" and which are "bad."

✔ All fats, even "good" fats, have a lot of calories, so you still need to limit them.

TYPES OF FAT

"Bad" Fats

- Saturated fat
- Trans fats or trans-fatty acids
- Hydrogenated fat
- Partially hydrogenated fat

"Good" Fats

- Unsaturated fat
- Polyunsaturated fat
- Monounsaturated fat
- Essential fats or essential fatty acids
- Omega-3 and omega-6 fatty acids

GOOD FATS

Good fats help to lower blood cholesterol if used in place of saturated fats. They tend to be liquid at room temperature. Here's how to use good fats in moderation:

- Use olive and canola oil (monounsaturated fats) for salads and cooking. (Cold-pressed oils are best, such as extra virgin cold-pressed olive oil.) If you cook with high heat, use peanut oil (it is more stable at high temperatures than most oils).

- Add good essential fatty acids, such as those found in flaxseed oil, to your diet. (Flaxseed oil must be refrigerated to prevent rancidity, and it cannot be heated. Flaxseed oil has a good taste if fresh.) Use flaxseed oil to extend "good-for-you" salad dressings. Add a teaspoon of flaxseed oil to two table-spoons of fat-free cream cheese and serve on a bagel! Add essential fats to your butter (if you use butter, use organic butter). Melt the butter, then add one part flaxseed oil to one part butter and refrigerate again until solid. (It tastes great!)

- Eat foods that contain monounsaturated fats, such as avocados, nuts, nut butters, and seeds. Fish like salmon and tuna also contain good fats.

Essential Fatty Acids (EFAs)

You need to add essential fatty acids to your diet because your body doesn't make them. Essential fatty acids include two types: omega-3 fatty acids and omega-6 fatty acids. Our bodies need EFAs in a ratio of about 3:1, omega-6 to omega-3, rather than the typical 20:1 ratio found in most diets. (The best way to do this is by supplementing your diet with omega-3 vegetable oils like flaxseed oil.)

Omega-6 fatty acids are found in oils such as corn oil, sunflower oil, safflower oil, and soybean oil. Other omega-6 fatty acid sources include black currant seed oil, borage oil, and evening primrose oil. Omega-3 fatty acids are found in foods such as flaxseeds, pumpkin seeds, walnuts, salmon, trout, and tuna. Flaxseed oil and hemp oil (both good tasting!) are the highest in omega-3 fatty acids.

BAD FATS

1. The worst "bad" fats are called trans fats (or trans-fatty acids). Trans fats are found in hydrogenated and partially hydrogenated oils. Trans fats raise the level of "bad" (LDL) cholesterol. In addition, trans fats lower the levels of "good" (HDL) cholesterol and raise the level of triglycerides (another form of blood fat linked to heart disease). Avoid these fats completely if you can. They are also linked to insulin resistance and have no redeeming health benefits!

Avoid trans fats by reading labels! Foods that almost always contain trans fats (hydrogenated or partially hydrogenated vegetable oils) include bake mixes, breads, cereals, margarines, salad dressings, snack foods, tortillas, and commercially prepared pies, cakes, and cookies, as well as other commercially prepared foods.

Avoid commercially prepared fried foods, such as fast-food French fries. These fried foods are high in trans fats.

Avoid trans fats by replacing margarine with a good fat product, such as Earth's Best Margarine (or another margarine containing no trans fats). Avoid trans fats by making your own salad dressings or by using low-fat dressings.

2. Another "bad" fat is saturated fat, which tends to be solid at room temperature. Saturated fats are found in animal products such as butter, cheese, whole milk, ice cream, cream, egg yolks, and fatty cuts of beef and pork. They are also found in some vegetable oils, such as coconut, palm, and palm kernel oils.

Saturated fat is linked to heart disease. However, it is not as harmful to the health as trans fats; saturated fats break down more easily in the body than trans fats. Nonetheless, avoid or reduce your intake of saturated fats. (If using saturated fat, the most healthful source is "organic"—from animals who are not given hormones or antibiotics.)

Cut back on saturated fat by cutting back on high-fat cuts of beef and pork, especially those found in fast food; they contain high levels of saturated fat.

Lower your at-home saturated fat consumption by trimming the fat from meats before you cook them and by using low-fat dairy products (such as low-fat milk and low-fat cheeses and yogurts). Reduce excess animal fat by removing the skin from chicken and turkey before you cook it.

Cook with olive oil or canola oil.

*Include essential fats like flaxseed oil
(but never heat them).*

*Avoid saturated fats and trans fats
(like hydrogenated and partially hydrogenated ones).*

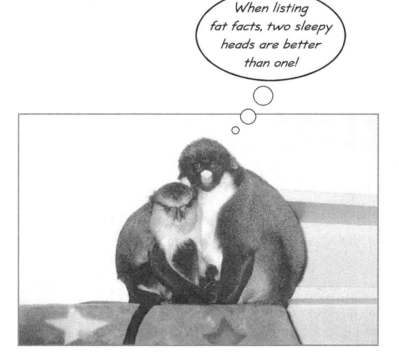

Molly's Good-Tasting Fiber-Rich Foods

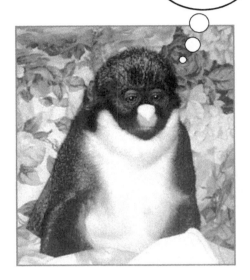

Just the fiber facts, please!

- Whole grains (like old-fashioned oatmeal and seven-grain bread)
- Nuts and seeds (like flaxseed meal, walnuts, cashews, almonds, sunflower seeds, and pumpkin seeds)
- Legumes, such as beans (including kidney beans, garbanzos, and lentils)
- Fruits (like strawberries, apples, blackberries, and blueberries)
- Veggies (like spaghetti squash, pea pods, artichokes, spinach, and broccoli)

THE FIBER FACTS

✔ Make fiber a part of each meal. It helps to slow the release of sugar into your body.

✔ Some fibers are soluble and some are insoluble. Both are important. Here's how fiber works: It remains mostly undigested in your gastrointestinal (GI) tract. This provides bulk to the foods you eat so that the undigested food stays in your stomach longer, making you feel fuller. Once in your intestine, it slows down the release of sugars and fats into your bloodstream. It helps blood sugar levels stay in control so less insulin is needed.

✔ Fiber makes you feel fuller, so you eat less without even thinking about it. Fiber is found in whole natural foods like veggies, fruits, grains, and legumes. Certain kinds of fiber can also be added to foods.

60

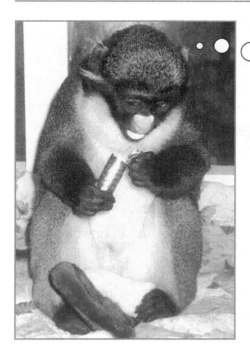

One for now! One for later!

✔ Some bland-tasting fibers you can sprinkle on your foods for added fiber include psyllium seed husk, guar gum, and oat bran.

✔ You can add fiber to meat or fish patties before cooking them by mixing oat or wheat bran into the mixture. Sprinkle flaxseed meal on cottage cheese and yogurt and use guar gum in protein drinks.

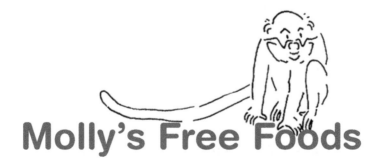

Molly's Free Foods

You do not need to include free foods in your calculations when they are eaten in moderation (one to two servings per meal). The keyword is "moderation." These foods are not totally calorie free. For example, if you consume eight servings of a free food (160 calories), it is equivalent to eating one English muffin.

Vegetables—Many vegetables are considered "free" foods, including celery, lettuce, spinach, cabbage, cucumbers, and zucchini. Free foods contain fewer than 20 calories per serving and less than 6 grams of carbohydrate per serving. These low-carb veggies have a high water content compared to most other free foods. When they are cooked, they lose the water and become more concentrated. For example, $\frac{1}{2}$ cup of raw free vegetables would have fewer calories than $\frac{1}{2}$ cup of cooked free vegetables. Therefore, cooked free vegetables have smaller portion sizes.

Drinks—Bouillon, broth, consommé, club soda, low-sodium diet soft drinks, sugar-free carbonated or mineral water, drink mixes, sugar-free cocoa powder (1 tablespoon), tea, coffee, and sugar-free tonic water

Flavorings, extracts, and spices—garlic, Tabasco or hot pepper sauce, fresh or dried herbs, wine (used in cooking), pimento, and Worcestershire sauce

Sugar-free or low-sugar foods—hard, sugar-free candy (one piece) (like the sugar-free mint Molly's having on page 61), gelatin dessert, sugar-free gelatin, unflavored gum, sugar-free jam or jelly, low-sugar or light syrup (2 teaspoons), sugar-free syrup (2 tablespoons)

Condiments—catsup (1 tablespoon), dill pickles (1$\frac{1}{2}$ large), horseradish, regular or light soy sauce, lemon juice, taco sauce (1 tablespoon), lime juice, vinegar, and mustard

Fat-free or reduced-fat foods—fat-free cream cheese (1 tablespoon), reduced-fat Miracle Whip (1 teaspoon), non-fat Miracle Whip (1 tablespoon), nondairy liquid creamers (1 tablespoon), nondairy powdered creamers (2 teaspoons), nonstick cooking spray, fat-free salad dressing (1 tablespoon), fat-free mayonnaise (1 tablespoon), reduced-fat mayonnaise (1 teaspoon), fat-free Italian salad dressing (2 tablespoons), salsa ($\frac{1}{4}$ cup), fat-free margarine (4 tablespoons), reduced-fat margarine (1 teaspoon), fat-free or reduced-fat sour cream (1 tablespoon), and regular or light whipped topping (2 tablespoons)

Nutrition Review

Q. What if I don't eat enough fiber-rich foods?

A. Sprinkle oat bran or another type of fiber on the foods you do eat.

Q. What if I have a meal without any low-carb veggies?

A. You will still need to balance your carbs, fruits, and high-carb veggies with an equal amount of protein!

DO . . .

1. Eat your protein food first (or at least part of it). Your fat and/or low-carb veggie foods can be eaten at the same time if you like. These foods digest in a way that does not make your blood sugar level go up quickly!

2. Then eat your high-carb veggies, legumes (these are high-carb beans and peas), or fruits. When these carbs mix with proteins in your stomach, they digest more slowly; therefore, sugar enters into your bloodstream more slowly.

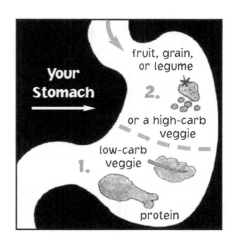

DON'T . . .

1. Don't eat your carb or fruits first! On an empty stomach, they can cause your blood sugar levels to go up rather quickly!

2. Don't skip the protein and eat only carbs! If you do, your blood sugar will go up rather quickly and then may get too low later! *This is NOT what you want!*

Molly's Fun Food-Planning List

Planning balanced meals will help keep your blood sugar levels even.

BASIC MEAL PLAN

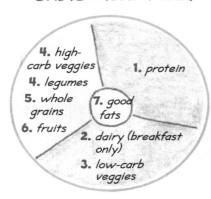

1. Proteins (no fiber): lean meats, lean cold cuts, lean fish, eggs and egg whites, egg substitutes, and tofu

2. Dairy foods (have some carbs and no fiber so are not interchangeable if counting carbs): low-fat milk, low-fat cheese, low-fat cottage or ricotta cheese, and low-fat sugar-free yogurt

3. Low-carb veggies (some fiber): lettuce, celery, tomato, cucumber, green beans, zucchini squash, summer squash, spaghetti squash, eggplant, spinach, parsley, cilantro, and bean sprouts

4. High-carb veggies (some fiber) and legumes (lots of fiber): Limit the amount of high-carb veggies: yellow winter squashes, yams, potatoes, sweet potatoes, beets, turnips, parsnips, and pumpkin. Legumes include kidney beans, garbanzo, navy beans, pinto beans, and dried peas like split peas and lentils.

5. Complex carbs or whole grains (high-fiber foods): old-fashioned oats, whole wheat, bulgur wheat, oat bran, whole rye, brown rice, quinoa, cornmeal, and whole-grain pasta

Breakfast

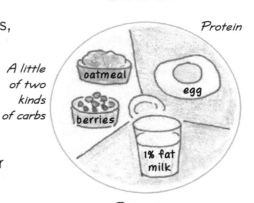

Lunch or Dinner

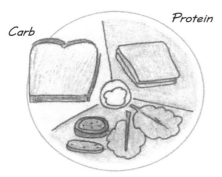

Carb

Protein

Low-carb veggies

6. Best fruit choices (some fiber—*all fruits have carbs*): strawberries, blue and black berries, acerola cherries, grapefruit, plums, and apples

7. Good fats (most have no fiber or are low in fiber): canola oil, olive oil, olives, raw nuts like walnuts, and fresh ground nut butters (no sugar). Flaxseed oil and flaxseed meal (high in fiber) taste good and are excellent sources of essential fatty acids.

More on Fine-Tuning Your Food Plan

Many people with diabetes are learning that it is most effective to watch their carbohydrate intake and to consult a glycemic index when choosing carbohydrate foods. This can be especially helpful for those who regularly have trouble keeping their blood sugar levels under control. (See page 99 for more about the glycemic index.)

Snack

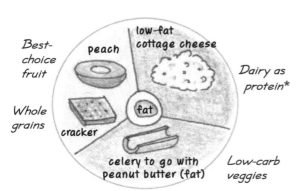

Best-choice fruit

peach

low-fat cottage cheese

Dairy as protein*

Whole grains

fat

cracker

celery to go with peanut butter (fat)

Low-carb veggies

*Consider mixing a spoonful of low-carb protein powder into dairy foods to give them a higher protein-to-carbohydrate ratio.

Lunch or Dinner

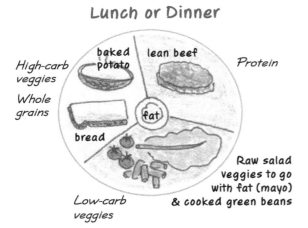

High-carb veggies
Whole grains
baked potato
lean beef
Protein
fat
bread
Low-carb veggies
Raw salad veggies to go with fat (mayo) & cooked green beans

Lunch or Dinner

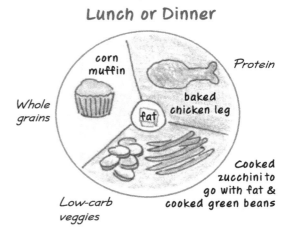

corn muffin
Protein
Whole grains
fat
baked chicken leg
Low-carb veggies
Cooked zucchini to go with fat & cooked green beans

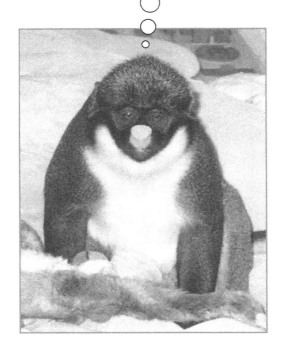

I'd like breakfast in bed, please!

Balance Second Helpings

Remember, overeating can make your blood sugar levels go up. Still, if you want second helpings of grains, high-carb veggies, or fruit, be sure to balance the second helping with protein, good fats, and low-carb veggies, as well!

Make balanced meals fun!

Molly's Favorite Protein-Balanced Recipes

These recipes are tasty, good for you, and easy to make! They have the benefit of being protein balanced. "Protein balanced" means that the protein and carbohydrates are pretty evenly balanced, which helps your blood sugar to stay more even.

PROTEIN-BALANCED FRUIT FRITTATAS

Makes 6 servings.

6 eggs

4 egg whites

½ cup 1% low-fat milk

4–6 packets of artificial sweetener

1 fragrant apple, with skin, cored and quartered

½ cup blueberries, fresh or frozen

½ cup low-fat cream cheese

2 tablespoons wheat germ

Nonstick cooking spray

1. Preheat the oven to 350°F. Blend eggs, egg white, milk, and sweetener in a blender or food processor. Add one-quarter of the apple at a time and blend. Add blueberries and blend. Add cream cheese and blend.

2. Coat a 9-x-9-inch glass baking dish with nonstick cooking spray. Pour in batter. Sprinkle top with wheat germ.

3. Bake for twenty minutes or until eggs are set. Frittata will rise as it bakes. *Wonderful!*

MOLLY'S PROTEIN-BALANCED FRENCH TOAST

Makes 2 pieces.

1 egg, beaten
1 cup 1-percent milk
2 slices of whole-grain bread
nonstick cooking spray, such as Pam

1. In a medium-sized bowl, mix egg with milk. Dip bread in mixture, covering both sides.

2. Brown coated bread over low heat in a nonstick skillet sprayed with nonstick cooking spray.

3. Serve with diet maple syrup and a glass of milk. *Heavenly!*

MOLLY'S PROTEIN-BALANCED OAT BRAN MUFFINS

Makes 2 small or 1 large muffin.

$\frac{1}{3}$ cup oat bran
$\frac{1}{3}$ cup low-fat ricotta cheese
1 egg
4–6 packets artificial sweetener
$\frac{1}{8}$ teaspoon vanilla or cinnamon
$\frac{1}{8}$ teaspoon baking powder

1. Preheat the oven to 350°F. Place all of the ingredients in a medium-sized mixing bowl. Mix well.

2. Spray two muffin spaces in a standard muffin pan with nonstick cooking spray. Pour in batter.

3. Bake for ten minutes until muffin springs back when you touch it. *Yummy!*

Microwave cooking: Place batter in a small microwave-safe dish. Cook on high for two minutes.

MOLLY'S MICROWAVE PROTEIN-BALANCED BLUEBERRY COOKIES

Makes 9 soft cookies.

$\frac{1}{3}$ cup applesauce

$\frac{1}{3}$ cup low-fat ricotta cheese

1 large egg

$\frac{1}{3}$ cup blueberries,
fresh or thawed and drained

$\frac{1}{3}$ cup Dr. Atkins low-carb bake mix
or soy flour

$\frac{1}{4}$ cup oat bran

10 packets artificial sweetener

1 teaspoon cinnamon

2 teaspoon baking powder

1. In a medium-sized mixing bowl, combine the applesauce, ricotta cheese, egg, and blueberries. Mix well.

2. Add the low-carb bake mix (or soy flour), oat bran, sweetener, cinnamon, and baking powder. Mix well.

3. Divide one-third of the batter into three parts and place about two inches apart on a microwave-safe plate.

4. Cook three cookies at a time in the microwave oven for approximately two minutes. Allow to cool before eating. *Delicious!*

Variation: For pancakes, add 1 tablespoon of water to the batter and spread out one-third of the batter to pancake size on a microwave-safe plate. Cook one pancake at a time in the microwave oven for approximately two minutes. Serve the pancakes with sugar-free syrup.

MOLLY'S PERFECT HIGH-FIBER PROTEIN-BALANCED HOT CEREAL

Makes 1 serving.

Cereal

3/4 cup dry oats

1 cup water

1 teaspoon cinnamon

1 heaping tablespoon flaxseed meal*

Artificial sweetener to taste (optional)

Do not heat flaxseed meal

Protein Milk

3/4 cup of low-fat milk

3/4 scoop of Jay Robb vanilla whey protein powder

1. Combine oats, water, and cinnamon in a microwave-safe bowl.

2. Cook for three to four minutes in the microwave oven until cereal is thickened and piping hot.

3. Remove from oven and sprinkle with flaxseed meal. (This gives you essential fatty acids and fiber.)

4. Stir in sweetener if desired. *Tasty!*

Conventional cooking: Combine oats, water, and cinnamon in a small pot. Cook over low heat for three to four minutes until cereal is thickened and piping hot. Remove from heat and stir in flaxseed meal. Stir in sweetener if desired.

Next, combine milk and protein powder. Blend in a blender or shake in a covered jar until frothy. Pour it over the hot cereal. *You will love it!*

"Good-for-You" Oil & Vinegar Dressing or Dip

Makes 6 tablespoons.

4 tablespoons vinegar

1 tablespoon olive oil

1 tablespoon flaxseed oil

1–2 teaspoons horseradish mustard or plain mustard

1–2 packets of artificial sweetener

Salt to taste

1. Blend together all of the ingredients. Chill.

2. Drizzle over a plain green salad or over a salad of chopped raw spinach, romaine, black kale, green and red onion, head lettuce, and parsley. *Delicious!*

Molly's Yogurt Salad Dressing or Dip

Makes 1 ¼ cups.

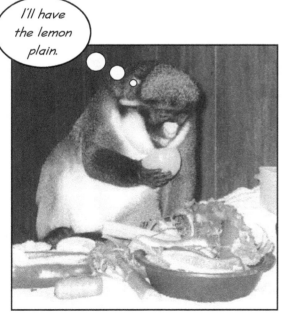

I'll have the lemon plain.

½ cup plain low-fat yogurt

½ cup sugar-free mayonnaise

Juice of one lemon or lime

½ to 1 tablespoon garlic salt, such as Lawry's
or ¼ package of onion soup mix, such as Lipton's

1. Combine all of the ingredients. Mix well. Chill.

2. Drizzle over salad or serve as a dip with low-carb veggies, such as raw celery sticks, bell pepper, and lightly cooked cauliflower and broccoli. *Yummy!*

Good Additions to Green Salads

🌶 Sprinkle salad with 1 tablespoon of seasoned pumpkin seeds or roasted soy nuts.

🌶 Spread ¼ cup of cooked green beans over salad.

🌶 Toss ¼ cup of chopped tomato and 1 tablespoon of chopped macadamia nuts into salad.

CUCUMBER & MAYONNAISE DRESSING OR DIP

Makes ¾ cup.

¼ cup sugar-free mayonnaise
¼ cup low-fat plain yogurt
⅓ cucumber, peeled
½ teaspoon garlic salt

1. Blend together all of the ingredients until the cucumber is liquefied. Chill.

2. Drizzle over green salad or serve as a dip with low-carb veggies, such as raw celery sticks, cauliflower, bell pepper, and broccoli.

Variation: For Tomato & Mayonnaise Dressing or Dip, replace the cucumber with one-quarter of a medium-sized tomato.

PROTEIN-BALANCED APPLE PIE SMOOTHIE

Makes 1 serving.

1¼ cup low-fat milk

³⁄₄ sliced raw apple

½ cup crushed ice

1 scoop Jay Robb's vanilla whey protein powder

1 teaspoon cinnamon

¼ teaspoon apple pie spice (optional)

½ to 1 teaspoon guar gum (optional)

1. Blend together milk, apple, and ice until smooth.

2. Add protein powder, cinnamon, apple pie spice (if desired), and guar gum (if desired). Blend until smooth.

This smoothie is so good, you won't believe it! It has lots of protein and fiber from the apple! YUM!

One of my favorite smart foods is a protein drink with good carbs and fiber. It's great tasting and it helps keep my blood sugar levels even.

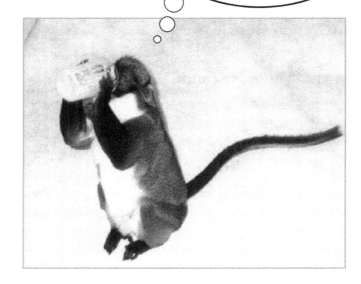

Food Products
Molly Recommends

The following are a few of the many products available that are tasty and nutritious and are smart choices for people with diabetes. *(Manufacturers' addresses and phone numbers are subject to change.)*

HIGH-PROTEIN, LOW-CARB BARS THAT TASTE LIKE CANDY

Keto Bar, Cookies N Cream

Nutrition Facts: 240 calories, 24 grams of protein, 4 grams of effective carbs, 6 grams of fat, and 4 grams of fiber.

Manufacturer: Life Services Supplements, Inc.
3535 Highway 66, Bldg. 2
Neptune, New Jersey 07753
1-800-542-3230

It's soft and cookie-like.

Peanut Butter Crunch Cookie

Nutrition Facts: 210 calories, 18 grams of protein, 8 grams of fat, 5 grams of fiber, and 0 grams of effective carbs.

Manufacturer: Pure De-Lite Products, Inc.
P.O. Box 50885
Provo, Utah 84605
1-866-4LO-CARB
www.puredelightproducts.com

Great-tasting cookie!

Nitro-Tech Peanut Butter Chocolate Chip Bar

Nutrition Facts: 35 grams of protein, 6 grams of carbs, 8 grams of fat, 4 grams of fiber.

Manufacturer: MuscleTech R & D Inc.
Mississauga, ON, Canada, L6W 4S6
1-800-246-3261

It's a delicious caramel-like bar with a chocolate coating.

Low Carb Lean Body Hi-Protein Meal Replacement Bar
(Chocolate Peanut Butter flavor and Pecan Pie flavor)

Nutrition Facts: 30 grams of protein, 2 grams of carbs, and 8 grams of fat.

Manufacturer: Labrada Nutrition
403 Century Plaza Dr., Suite 440
Houston TX 77073
1-800-832-9948

It's delicious.

Myoplex Low Carb Bar
(Blueberry, Lemon Cheesecake, Apple Cinnamon)

Nutrition Facts: 28 grams of protein, 3.5 grams of carbs, and 6 grams of fat.

Manufacturer: EAS, Inc.
555 Corporate Circle
Golden CO 80401
1-800-297-9776

Ultimate Lo-Carb 2 Bar
(Chocolate Smores Supreme)

Nutrition Facts: 3 grams of carbs, 20 grams of protein, and 6 grams of fat.

Manufacturer: Biochem Sports and Fitness Systems (a division of Country Life)
101 Corporate Drive
Hauppauge, NY 11788
1-800-645-5768

Doctor's Lo-Carb Diet Bar

(Chocolate Covered Banana Nut flavor)

Nutrition Facts: 21 grams of protein, 2 grams of carbohydrate, and 4 grams of fat.

Manufacturer: Universal Nutrition
3 Terminal Road
New Brunswick, NJ 08901
1-800-USA-0101 or
1-800-872-0101

Atkins Advantage Bar

Nutrition Facts: 250 calories, 2 grams of carbs, 19 grams of protein, and 5 grams of fiber.

Manufacturer: Atkins Nutritionals, Inc.
2002 Orville Drive North, Suite A
Ronkonkoma, NY 11779
1-800-6ATKINS

The chocolate peanut butter bar is great tasting!

OTHER PRODUCTS

Fiber-Rich Bagels, Cinnamon Raisin

Nutrition Facts: (1/2 bagel): 45 calories, 4 grams of protein, 10 grams of carb, 1 gram of fat, and 7 grams of fiber.

Manufactured for: Controlled Carb Gourmet
8780 Charleston Blvd., Suite 193
Las Vegas, NV 89117
1-800-598-7720
www.controlledcarbgourmet.com

Delicious!

Jay Robb Hormone-Free Whey Protein Powder
(Strawberry, Vanilla, Chocolate)

Manufacturer: Jay Robb Enterprises Inc.
1530 Encinitas Blvd.
Encinitas, CA 92024
1-877-JAYROBB

This is the best-tasting whey protein powder I've ever had!
Be sure to try Jay Robb egg white protein powder, too!

Atkin's Bake Mix

Nutrition Facts ($\frac{1}{4}$ cup serving): 18 grams of protein, 6 grams of carbs, and 2 grams of fat.

Manufacturer: Atkins Nutritionals Inc.
2002 Orville Drive North, Suite A
Ronkonkoma, NY 11779
1-800-6ATKINS

PART THREE

Diabetes in Depth

Understanding Diabetes

Diabetes is a chronic, complex disorder. It is characterized by the inability to properly metabolize blood sugar (glucose). Glucose metabolism is regulated by the hormone insulin, which allows cells to use glucose from the bloodstream. Without insulin, glucose levels build up in the blood and in the urine while the cells starve for nourishment. People with either type 1 or type 2 diabetes must control their blood sugar or risk serious health consequences. In both forms of diabetes, high levels of blood sugar for extended periods of time can cause injury to many organs and tissues. The better you do now at keeping your blood sugar level even, the less likely you are to have serious health problems later.

THE DIFFERENCES BETWEEN TYPE 1 AND TYPE 2 DIABETES

Type 1 Diabetes

- Type 1 diabetes is also known as juvenile diabetes. This is because it occurs most often in children and young adults.

- Type 1 diabetes accounts for 5 to 10 percent of people with diabetes.

- Type 1 diabetes is an autoimmune disease in which the insulin-producing islets of the pancreas are destroyed by a malfunctioning immune system. As you've learned, the body uses insulin to keep blood sugar at a safe and constant level. There are no oral medications that can restore the insulin-producing islets. Once the islets are dead, the body needs insulin from an outside source.

- The treatment for type 1 diabetes includes daily insulin injections (sometimes several injections depending on the individual's condition) and careful dietary monitoring.

- People with type 1 diabetes can better control their blood sugar and stay healthier by doing the following:

  - Taking prescribed medication (knowing how quickly your insulin works and taking insulin injections as needed)

  - Meal planning (eating healthy balanced meals and knowing how quickly you metabolize different foods)

  - Exercising (having a regular, doctor supervised exercise regimen, preferably exercising every day, but if not, every other day)

  - Self-monitoring (using blood glucose meters and test strips to check blood sugar levels as needed throughout the day and keeping weight under control)

  - Joining diabetes support groups (members sharing common experiences and problems can help relieve stress and may also help with ongoing education)

  - Maintaining ongoing education (keeping up with the latest products and treatments for people with type 1 diabetes may alert you to new options)

Hard-to-control factors include anything that may influence your blood sugar levels such as stress, irregular mealtimes, unplanned activity or exercise, illness (the flu, nausea, vomiting, or diarrhea may interfere with your regular meals), lack of sleep, and irregular timing of injections.

Type 2 Diabetes

- Type 2 diabetes is a metabolic disorder. It is the result of insulin resistance combined with beta cell (pancreatic islet cells that secrete insulin) fatigue or failure.

- People over age forty who are overweight and sedentary (inactive) are at risk for developing type 2 diabetes.

- Type 2 diabetes usually occurs in older people, but it is increasingly becoming a problem in younger adults and children. It accounts for 90 to 95 percent of people with diabetes.

- Because the insulin-producing islets are still alive, people with type 2 diabetes may sometimes be able to manage their disease by doing the following:
  - keeping their weight under control
  - eating balanced meals
  - exercising regularly
  - reducing stress levels
- People with type 2 diabetes can also benefit from taking one or more oral medications prescribed by their doctors.
- An estimated 40 percent of people with type 2 diabetes may require insulin injections, sometimes along with oral medications.
- People with type 2 diabetes who use insulin may become increasingly insensitive to it. This is known as insulin sensitivity or insulin resistance.
- People with type 2 diabetes can improve insulin sensitivity and help prevent diabetes-related health problems by doing the following:
  - eating balanced meals
  - drinking little or no alcohol
  - exercising regularly (weight resistance exercise and aerobics appear to be the most beneficial for improving insulin resistance)
  - not smoking
  - reducing stress

Insulin and Oral Medications

INSULIN USERS . . .

Ideally, both diabetes patients and their doctors will develop an overview of, first, how insulin and diabetes medications work and, second, of what types of insulin and oral medications are available. This helps the patient and doctor to work well together and aids people with diabetes in participating more in the journey of their own care.

COMBINATION THERAPY FOR TYPE 2 DIABETES

For those with type 2 diabetes who require insulin injections, combination therapy means the use of insulin combined with the use of oral medications for better glucose level control.

Also, using combination therapy may permit fewer insulin injections. Few insulin injections can be a psychological relief and, therefore, can improve a person's willingness to comply with overall prescribed care.

TYPE 1 OR TYPE 2—WHICH INSULIN IS RIGHT FOR YOU?

One or more types of insulin can be taken to manage blood sugar levels. People with diabetes don't respond to individual types or amounts of insulin the same way. By working with your doctor or healthcare team, you can find the right insulin (or insulin combination) in the amount that works for your eating and exercise patterns.

Types of Insulin

There are more than twenty types of insulin products available in four basic forms, each with a different time of onset and duration of action. The decision about which insulin to choose is based on an individual's lifestyle, a physician's preference and experience, and the person's blood sugar levels. Among the criteria considered in choosing insulin are:

- how soon it starts working (onset)
- when it works the hardest (peak time)
- how long it lasts in the body (duration)

Very Fast-Acting Insulin

- **Lispro and aspart:** The fastest acting insulins require a prescription. They are called lispro (Humalog) and insulin aspart (Novolog). They can be used before meals to help keep post-meal blood sugar (often elevated in those with diabetes) from rising too high. These insulins should be injected under the skin within fifteen minutes before you eat. You have to remember to eat within fifteen minutes after you take a shot. These insulins start working in five to fifteen minutes and lower your blood sugar most in forty-five to ninety minutes. They finish working in three to four hours. With regular insulin, you have to wait thirty to forty-five minutes before eating. Many people like using lispro because it's easier to coordinate eating with this type of insulin.

Fast-acting (or regular) Insulin

- Fast-acting insulin is also called regular insulin. It is considered a short-acting insulin and lowers blood sugar most in two to five hours and finishes its work in five to eight hours.

Intermediate Acting Insulin

- **NPH (N) or Lente (L):** These insulins start working in one to three hours, lower your blood sugar most in six to twelve hours and finish working in twenty to twenty-four hours.

Other Insulins

- **Human Ultralente:** Has a longer duration of activity than Lente or NPH.
- **Glargine:** Taken only once a day at bedtime. It can be used with a very-rapid-acting insulin such as lispro or aspart, and should provide a longer, steadier release of insulin. Until now, this has only been possible with twice daily

injections of Ultralente or by the basal rate of an insulin pump. This approach tries to permit more normal mealtime patterns individualized to a person's own habits.

- **Aspart:** A very-rapid-acting insulin that can be injected 15 minutes prior to eating. Its fast action also allows more freedom in the timing of meals and the amount of food eaten.

Insulin Mixtures

- **Humalog Mix 75:** A combination of Humalog and NPL (also 70/30).

- A 75/25 lispro mixture is the first of the analog mixtures available (from Eli Lilly); it contains Lilly's very-rapid-acting lispro and a novel human insulin analog called NPL. It is designed for those who need better control after meals and want to use an insulin pen.

Insulin Type	Action Begins	Peak	Duration
Humalog®	5 minutes	1 hour	2–4 hours
Regular	15–30 minutes	2–4 hours	4–6 hours
NPH	30–60 minutes	4–8 hours	20–22 hours
Lente	60 minutes	9–12 hours	22–24 hours
Ultralente®	1–2 hours	9–15 hours	24–26 hours
Lantus®	1.1 hours	no pronounced peak	24+ hours

Insulin Storage

- If you use a whole bottle of insulin within thirty days, you can safely keep it at room temperature.

- If you don't use a whole bottle within thirty days, you should keep it in the refrigerator all of the time.

- If insulin gets too hot or too cold, it doesn't work right. So don't let your insulin freeze or overheat.

- Store at least one extra bottle of insulin in your refrigerator.

Ways to Administer Insulin

Insulin is not available in oral form because it would be destroyed by acids in the stomach. Many research efforts are currently aimed at developing easier ways to use insulin. It is now administered as follows:

Syringe—Using a syringe, injectable insulin must be injected under the skin (as recommended by your doctor to keep your blood sugar levels even).

Jet injector—Jet injectors use pressure to "push" the insulin into the skin. They send a fine spray of insulin through the skin using a high-pressure air mechanism instead of needles. These are good for people who fear needles; however, they are expensive, and you have to boil and sterilize the units frequently.

Insulin pen—Insulin pens function similarly to syringes but contain pre-filled cartridges and look like a cartridge pen. These are handy if you want the convenience of carrying insulin with you in a discreet way. Some pens use replaceable cartridges of insulin and other models are disposable. The tip of the pen has a fine, short needle. Users turn a dial to select the desired dose of insulin and press a plunger on the end to deliver the insulin.

External insulin pump—The insulin pump connects to plastic tubing that ends with a needle inserted just under the skin near the abdomen. It is lightweight and small, about the size of a deck of cards and can be worn on a belt or in a pocket. Users set the pump to give them a steady amount of insulin continuously throughout the day. Pumps can release several doses of insulin at a time, at meals and at times when blood sugar levels are too high. If you use an insulin pump, it's very important to monitor your blood sugar frequently so you can determine the right dose and also to be sure that the insulin is being delivered.

Where Should You Inject?

You can inject insulin into several places on your body. Insulin injected near the stomach works fastest. Insulin injected into the thigh works slowest, and a shot in the arm works at medium speed. Again, work with your doctor regarding the area you will use for injection and to make sure you are injecting the insulin properly.

ORAL MEDICATIONS FOR TYPE 2 DIABETES

Oral medications work best in people with type 2 diabetes who have had high blood sugar for less than ten years and who have normal weight. It's not uncommon for oral medication to control blood sugar well for years and then stop working. When one type of oral medication stops working, another may be tried with success. Some individuals who return to the first medication at a later time find it works again. In some people, taking more than one oral medication may work better than taking either one alone. Some people who begin treatment with oral medications eventually need to take insulin.

Sulfonylureas

These are a class of medications that act to force the pancreas to release more insulin, which then lowers your blood sugar. For this medication to work, your pancreas has to make some insulin. If your pancreas makes no insulin at all, you are not a good candidate for sulfonylureas. Also, if you have an allergy to sulfa drugs, you should probably avoid sulfonylureas.

This class of drugs includes chlorpropamide (Diabinese), glyburide (DiaBeta, Micronase, Glynase), glipizide (Glucotrol), glimepiride (Amaryl), and tolbutamide.

Some sulfonylureas work all day; therefore, you take them only once. Other types are taken twice each day. Your doctor will tell you how many times a day you should be taking your sulfonylurea.

These are potent, effective, and have relatively few side effects, but can cause weight gain, an upset stomach, skin rash or itching, and low blood sugar. Over time, they may lose their effectiveness. Amaryl can be used alone or with insulin. These drugs should not be used by anyone with liver problems and should be used with caution by older people. Diabinese should not be used by people with kidney problems.

Biguanides

- **Metformin (Glucophage and Glucophage XR):** This medication is known as a biguanide. It helps keep the blood sugar from climbing too high by preventing the formation and release of sugar in the liver. Metformin also lowers the amount of insulin in your body. You may lose a few pounds when you start to take metformin. This weight loss can help you control your blood glucose. Metformin can also improve blood fat and cholesterol levels, which are often high if you have type 2 diabetes. It can be used alone or with insulin.

  Metformin is taken two to three times each day with a meal; your doctor will tell you which meals to take it with. Glucophage XR is the long-acting version of Glucophage. (Your doctor will advise you on whether or not it might help you and on how to take it.)

  Metformin should not be used by people who drink more than about two to four alcoholic drinks a week. If you drink more than that, this medication will make you sick. Do not take metformin if you have liver or kidney problems (make sure your doctor checks your kidneys before putting you on this medication, since it can build up in your system if your kidneys aren't functioning properly). Other potential side effects include bloating, gassiness, diarrhea, nausea, and a metallic taste in your mouth.

Alpha-Glucosidase Inhibitors

- **Acarbose (Precose)** and **miglitol (Glyset)** are known as alpha-glucosidase inhibitors. They normalize post-meal blood sugar levels by slowing carbohydrate absorption (both medications block the enzymes that digest the starches you eat). This action causes a slower and lower rise of blood sugar through the day, but mainly right after meals.

  Acarbose and miglitol should be taken with the first bite of a meal. They are taken three times daily, at mealtime, although your doctor might ask you to take the medication less often at first.

  People with kidney problems should not use these drugs. To decrease the likelihood of side effects like gassiness and bloating, users may start with a low dose and increase it over a few weeks. Do not use digestive enzyme supplement products like Beano. They will stop the action. Stomach problems such as gas, bloating, and diarrhea often go away after you take the medication for a while.

Thiazolidinediones

The medication works by helping to make your cells more sensitive to insulin. The insulin can then move glucose from your blood into your cells for energy. You may take a thiazolidinedione as your only medication, or your doctor may ask you to take another diabetes medication along with it.

- **Rosiglitazone (Avandia)** and **pioglitazone (Actos)**: These seek to resensitize the body to insulin and improve blood sugar levels.

  Rosiglitazone is taken either once or twice a day, at the same time each day, usually in the morning, with or without a meal; or in the morning and in the evening, with or without meals. Pioglitazone is usually taken once a day at the same time, with or without a meal.

  People taking these medications should have liver tests every other month for a year, then periodically afterward. Call your doctor immediately if you develop any signs of liver disease, which include nausea, vomiting, stomach pain, lack of appetite, tiredness, yellowing of the skin or whites of the eyes, or dark-colored urine. People with liver problems should not take these medications. Take with caution if used with insulin or other diabetes medications; your blood sugar might drop too low. Weight gain, anemia, and swelling in the legs or ankles are also possible side effects.

Meglitinides

- **Repaglinide (Prandin)**: This medication causes the pancreas to release more insulin right after meals, so helps to reduce high blood sugar. Replagninide is both fast-acting and short-acting (it works fast and your body uses it quickly) and is usually taken three times a day before meals. This fast action means you can vary the times you eat and the number of meals you eat more easily than you can with other diabetes medications. If it doesn't work alone to control your blood sugar levels, your doctor might recommend that you try it with another medication like metformin.

Repaglinide is taken from thirty minutes before to just before a meal. It lowers blood sugar the most one hour after it's taken, and it is out of the bloodstream in three to four hours. If you skip a meal, you shouldn't take the dose.

This drug should be used with caution in people with liver problems. Side effects may include hypoglycemia (low blood sugar), weight gain, gastrointestinal discomfort, and sinus problems.

Other Oral Medications

- **Nateglinide (Starlix):** This medication is a derivative of the amino acid phenylalanine. It's taken before meals to normalize post-meal blood sugar levels. Starlix can be used on its own or taken in combination with metformin.

- **Glucovance:** This is a tablet that combines glyburide and metformin. It is one of the medications that your doctor might try initially (along with a healthy diet and exercise) to try to better manage your blood sugar levels. It's also recommended for people whose blood sugar can't be controlled by taking either sulfonylurea or metformin alone.

Nutritional Supplements

Supplements taken by some people with diabetes include vitamins, minerals, antioxidants, bioflavonoids, herbs, amino acids, and essential fats. Many of these alternative nutritional therapies have proven their value and have become accepted by healthcare professionals (especially when taken in sufficient amounts). There are some, however, that remain unproven.

Most experts agree the first line of defense in diabetes care should be to control your blood sugar by following your exercise and meal plan and using the proven, effective medications your doctor has prescribed. While supplements have been shown to provide health benefits to people with both type 1 and type 2 diabetes, it's important *not* to think of them as magic pills that will substitute for first-line care!

Consult your doctor or diabetes healthcare team before making any changes in your self care.

MINERALS

Chromium picolinate supplements have been found to improve insulin's efficiency, which lowers blood sugar levels. It improves glucose tolerance in people with both type 1 and type 2 diabetes (apparently by increasing sensitivity to insulin). Chromium also improves the processing of glucose in women with gestational diabetes. Chromium supplements have been shown to decrease fasting glucose levels, improve glucose tolerance, lower insulin levels, and decrease LDL ("bad") cholesterol and triglyceride levels, while increasing HDL ("good") cholesterol levels. Niacin administered at relatively low levels along with chromium has been shown to be more effective than chromium alone.

Magnesium levels are found to be significantly lowered in people with diabetes, and lowest levels are found in those with severe retinopathy. A deficiency of magnesium in people with type 2 diabetes may interrupt insulin secretion in the pancreas and increase insulin resistance in the body's tissues. Therefore, a deficiency in magnesium may worsen the blood sugar control in type 2 diabetes. Supplementation with magnesium leads to improved insulin production in elderly people with type 2 diabetes. When people with type 1 diabetes supplement with magnesium, insulin requirements are found to be lower. Studies show that in magnesium-deficient people with type 1 diabetes, diabetes-induced eye damage is more likely to occur.

Vanadium, which is found in small amounts in plants and animals, aids insulin's ability to move glucose into the cells. In the form of vanadyl sulfate, it has been shown to normalize blood glucose levels in animals with both type 1 and type 2 diabetes. In a human study, people who took vanadium in the form of vanadyl sulfate developed a modest increase in insulin sensitivity and were able to decrease their insulin requirements. It appears most efficient when used in conjunction with chromium and other vitamins and minerals that work synergistically to help regulate blood sugar levels and correct deficiencies. Use with your physician's supervision only.

Manganese deficiency in animals was found to result in diabetes. People with type 2 diabetes have been found to have only one-half the manganese of normal individuals. Manganese plays an important role in glucose metabolism.

Potassium supplementation has been shown to yield improved insulin sensitivity, plus improved insulin responsiveness and secretion in people with type 2 diabetes. Insulin administration often causes a potassium deficiency.

Zinc is involved in all aspects of insulin metabolism—synthesis, secretion, and utilization. People with type 1 diabetes tend to be zinc deficient, which may also impair immune function. Zinc supplements have lowered blood sugar levels in people with type 1 diabetes. People with type 2 diabetes also have low zinc levels, caused by excess loss of zinc in their urine. Use zinc gluconate lozenges for best absorption.

VITAMINS

Vitamin C deficiency may lead to vascular problems in people with diabetes. Vitamin C may slow or help prevent complications that occur in people with diabetes. Vitamin C helps lower sorbitol (a sugar that can accumulate and damage the eyes, nerves, and kidneys of people with diabetes). Vitamin C may improve glucose tolerance in people with type 2 diabetes. Low levels of vitamin C have been found in people with type 1 diabetes.

Vitamin E improves insulin activity and acts as an antioxidant and a blood oxygenator. Research has shown that people with low blood levels of vitamin E are more likely to develop type 2 diabetes. People with diabetes have been shown to have a higher than usual need for vitamin E. Double-blind studies show that vitamin E improves glucose tolerance in people with type 2 diabetes. Vitamin E may help prevent diabetic complications through its antioxidant activity and the inhibition of the platelet-releasing reaction and platelet aggregation, increasing HDL cholesterol levels and its role in fatty acid metabolism. Use the d-alpha-tocopherol form.

Vitamin B$_6$ (pyridoxine) has been shown to be deficient in people who have diabetic neuropathy (nerve damage caused by diabetes). Such people have been shown to benefit from vitamin B$_6$ supplementation. Vitamin B$_6$ supplements also improve glucose tolerance in women with gestational diabetes.

Vitamin B$_{12}$ is needed for normal functioning of nerve cells; it has been shown to help prevent diabetic neuropathy. Vitamin B$_{12}$ supplementation has been used with some success in treating diabetic neuropathy. Vitamin B$_{12}$ has been taken orally or by doctor-supervised injection to reduce nerve damage caused by diabetes. If taken orally, use a lozenge or sublingual form.

Biotin is a B vitamin that improves the metabolism of glucose in people with diabetes. Biotin may also reduce pain from diabetic nerve damage.

Niacin is a form of vitamin B$_3$ that can benefit people with diabetes if supplemented in small amounts *but not in large amounts.* Daily supplementation with 2–3 grams of niacin has been shown to *impair* glucose tolerance. Smaller amounts of niacin (500–750 mg per day for one month followed by 250 mg per day) may help some people with type 2 diabetes. Another form of niacin, called niacinamide, has been shown to slow down the destruction of insulin-producing beta cells in the pancreas, as well as to enhance their regeneration. Niacinamide may be helpful for people with both type 1 and type 2 diabetes.

Inositol is important for circulation and to prevent atherosclerosis. Inositol is needed in the body for normal nerve function. Some cases of nerve damage or diabetic neuropathy caused by diabetes have been reversed by inositol supplementation.

ADDITIONAL SUPPLEMENTS

Alpha-lipoic acid (ALA) is a powerful natural antioxidant that has been used for treatment of peripheral nerve damage in patients with diabetes. It has also been shown to help control blood sugar levels. In several studies, ALA has been used to improve diabetic neuropathies and has reduced pain.

Coenzyme Q_{10} (CoQ$_{10}$) improves circulation and stabilizes blood sugar. CoQ_{10} is needed to aid in normal carbohydrate metabolism in people with diabetes. Animals with diabetes have been found to be CoQ_{10} deficient. In a human trial, blood sugar levels of people with diabetes fell substantially in one-third of the cases after they supplemented with CoQ_{10}. CoQ_{10} is an antioxidant that fights free-radical damage and is a blood oxygenator. Because the eye is so richly supplied with tiny blood vessels, CoQ_{10} can help in cases of retinopathy.

Quercetin has been shown to help protect the lens of the eye from accumulations of polyols that result from chronic high blood sugar levels.

Alpha-lipoic acid and coenzyme Q_{10} are antioxidants. Antioxidants are natural compounds that help protect the body from harmful free radicals (atoms or groups of atoms that can cause damage to cells). Quercetin is a bioflavonoid. Although bioflavonoids are not considered true vitamins, they are sometimes referred to as vitamin P.

ESSENTIAL FATTY ACIDS

Gamma-linolenic acid (GLA) is a fatty acid found in black currant seed oil, borage oil, and evening primrose oil. GLA has been shown to be helpful for improving damaged nerve function, which is common in diabetes. Supplementing with evening primrose oil has been found to reverse diabetic nerve damage and lower cholesterol in people with both type 1 and type 2 diabetes.

AMINO ACIDS

Amino acids are found in protein-rich foods. Take them with water on an empty stomach at least a half hour before eating protein foods. Take them with vitamin C for better absorption.

L-carnitine is an amino acid needed by the body to properly use fat for energy. Carnitine improves the breakdown of fatty acids, possibly playing a role in preventing diabetic ketoacidosis.

L-glutamine is an amino acid that can help reduce sugar cravings.

Taurine is an amino acid that can aid in the release of insulin in people with type 2 diabetes. People with type 1 diabetes have low taurine levels, which can lead to "thickened" blood (a condition that increases the risk of heart disease).

HERBS

Herbs have been used for centuries in some countries to help lower blood sugar levels in people with type 2 diabetes. Not all herbal products are standardized. Many herbs have been used with reported success, including *Gymnema sylvestre,* fenugreek, bitter melon (extracts of fruits and not seeds, leaves, or any other parts of the vine), and garlic (has been shown to decrease blood sugar levels, to stabilize blood sugar levels, and to improve circulation).

PART FOUR

The Glycemic Index

An Introduction to the Glycemic Index (GI)

The glycemic index (GI) is a way of classifying the carbohydrates we eat (such as rice, cereal, potato, or pasta) according to their effect on blood sugar. High GI foods are foods that digest rapidly, leading to a fast release of glucose into your bloodstream. Low GI foods are foods that digest more slowly, releasing glucose into your bloodstream gradually.

The GI is of special importance to people with diabetes. It can help you make better carbohydrate selections: eating lower GI foods means a slower, smaller elevation of blood sugar. Therefore, less insulin (or type 2 diabetes medication) is needed to bring blood sugar levels under control.

MAKING CARB CHOICES

Although simple sugars (such as table sugar, honey, fruit sugar, and milk sugar) sometimes have a higher GI than complex carbs (such as breads, potatoes, peas, corn, legumes, rice, and pasta), this is not always the case. Complex carbs can be high GI (such as baked potato and puffed brown rice), and simple sugars can be low GI (such as blueberries and strawberries).

GENERAL GI GUIDELINES

GIs are compiled by testing groups of people. Single foods are fed to each individual on an empty stomach. When more than one food is combined in a meal or snack, many factors influence the overall GI of that meal or snack (thereby lowering the effective GI). These factors include the following:

- The amount of fiber in a meal—fiber slows down the digestion of starches in the intestine (juices, for example, always have a higher GI than the foods they are made from, simply because the fiber is missing).

- The amount of protein in a meal—protein slows the rate of stomach emptying and slows the digestive rate in the intestines.

- The amount of fat in a meal—like protein, fat slows the rate of stomach emptying and slows the digestive rate in the intestines (but too much fat is harmful to the health and it should not be overeaten).

- Particle size—finely milled grain (such as wheat flour or oat flour) will digest faster than whole-grain particles (such as roughly milled whole wheat, wheat berries, and whole oats).

- The type of starch in your food—foods like legumes and basmati rice have a greater amount of a starch called amylose when compared to the amount of one called amylopectin (amylose lowers the speed of the starch digestion).

- Whether foods are raw or cooked—cooking breaks down fiber, causing some cooked foods to absorb faster than raw or lightly cooked ones. Some GI lists include only foods prepared in one way and do not indicate whether they were tested raw or cooked (cooked carrots, for example, are rated high and raw carrots are rated low, but often only "carrots" is listed). Cooking also changes the starch in some foods, causing it to swell and therefore to absorb faster in the intestines—the less swelling, the slower the digestive rate.

A simple tomato can be helpful, eh?

- The acidity of foods—high acid foods, such as vinegar, citrus fruit, or tomato slow down the rate of digestion when added to your meals.

USE COMMON SENSE

Don't let the GI be the only factor you consider in choosing your foods. Some high GI foods are better nutritional choices than some low GI foods. For example, high GI cooked carrots are more nutritious than high-fat ice cream or high-fat fudge, which are low GI.

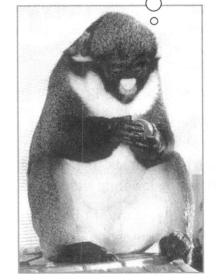

MEALTIME GI REVIEW

- Although low GI fruits and vegetables are
  the best choice, higher-glycemic carbs
  can be combined with lower GI carbs (for
  example, in the carb section of your plate,
  serve half a portion of high GI baked potato with
  half a portion of lower GI peas). Also, when you eat
  high GI carbs as part of a balanced meal, you will also
  be combining them with protein, low-carb veggies,
  and appropriate amounts of fat. This will produce
  a lower GI response for your overall meal or snack.

*Remember...
Using lower GI foods
in a meal will reduce
the overall GI of
that meal!*

- Be aware that many common manufactured foods and junk foods have a low
  GI because they are high in fat. French-fried potatoes and potato chips (high
  in "bad" fats), have a lower GI than a plain baked potato. However, the GI of
  a baked potato could be lowered with 2 teaspoons of "good" fat on top (and
  by eating it as part of a balanced meal with protein and a green salad). Such
  a choice would be much more healthful than the high "bad fat" fries or chips.

- The mixed-ingredient food GI equation: a combination of ingredients in a
  recipe (like a muffin baked with egg, milk, flour, oats, bran, and blueberries)
  works the same way as eating different GI foods in a meal. Lower glycemic
  ingredients help bring down the GI of the finished product.

**The Mealtime
GI Equation**

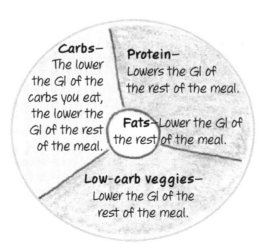

Carbs—
The lower
the GI of the
carbs you eat,
the lower the
GI of the rest
of the meal.

Protein—
Lowers the GI of
the rest of the meal.

Fats—Lower the GI of
the rest of the meal.

Low-carb veggies—
Lower the GI of the
rest of the meal.

Why do some glycemic index lists give different numbers for the same foods?

Glycemic index lists assign a numerical value to a food, which indicates how much and how rapidly its carb content will raise blood sugar levels when compared with a reference food (usually glucose or white bread). The reference food is given an arbitrary value of 100.

Different GI lists give different numbers for the same foods for a variety of reasons. For example, people as individuals have different levels of sensitivity to carbs and, therefore, a different range of responses. When a group is tested to determine GI values, the individual reactions to a given food are then averaged. As individuals, our reactions may be different from the average. Other reasons that GI lists give different numbers can inlcude: different length cooking times and different degrees of ripeness of fruit, and so on.

It is useful for people with diabetes to know how quickly they metabolize different foods; by providing a general guideline, *the GI is the most effective tool so far in helping achieve this goal.* It helps those of us with diabetes to adjust insulin or oral medications to more closely match what we eat (to help keep our blood sugar levels more even).

GI HEALTH BENEFITS REVIEW

- Low GI foods lead to more even blood glucose levels following a meal or snack than do high GI foods.

- Low GI diets have been reported to lead to improved insulin responses and better blood lipid profiles (for example, improved blood cholesterol).

- Because the carbohydrate is absorbed slowly from low GI foods, in some cases they can help in weight control by delaying the return of feelings of hunger.

Molly's Glycemic Index List

Glycemic Index Standard = 100%   (White bread)

Glycemic Index greater than 100% (Very High Range)

- Corn flakes
- Fat-free baguette
- Fat-free French bread
- Glucose

- Hot-air popcorn (fat free)
- Instant potato
- Instant white rice
- Maltose

- Millet
- Puffed millet
- Puffed rice
- Puffed rice cakes

- Puffed wheat
- Refined cereals (most)
- Rice Krispies
- Tofu non-dairy ice cream

Glycemic Index between 80% and 100% (High Range)

- Apricots (ripe)
- Baked potato
- Banana (ripe or overripe)
- Barley (cooked)
- Brown rice
- Buckwheat flour
- Carrots (cooked)
- Coarse ground wheat

- Corn
- Corn chips
- Grapenuts
- Honey
- Ice cream (low fat)
- Instant mashed potatoes
- Mango (ripe)
- Muesli

- Oat bran (cooked)
- Oat flour
- Papaya (ripe)
- Parsnips
- Popcorn (oil popped)
- Quick-cooking oats
- Raisins

- Rolled oats
- Rye flour
- Shredded wheat
- Watermelon
- White rice
- Whole-wheat bread

Glycemic Index between 40% and 79% (Moderate Range)**

- All-Bran cereal
- Apple juice
- Applesauce
- Baked beans
- Barley
- Bran
- Butter beans
- Cooked beets
- Cooked tomato
- Cooked winter squash
- Couscous
- Grapes
- Kidney beans
- Lima beans
- Navy or white beans
- Old-fashioned oats
- Onion
- Orange juice
- Oranges
- Pasta noodles
- Pears
- Peas
- Pinto beans
- Pumpernickel bread
- Raisins
- Spaghetti (white flour)
- Spaghetti (whole wheat)
- Split peas
- Steel-cut oats
- Sweet potato
- Wheat berries (kernels)
- Whole-grain rye
- Yam

Glycemic Index 40% or less (Low Range)

- Apples (pippin especially)
- Banana (under-ripe)
- Berries (such as strawberries, blueberries, and black berries)
- Black-eyed peas
- Broccoli
- Cabbage
- Carrot (raw)
- Cauliflower
- Celery
- Chana dal (bean)
- Cherries (sour)
- Cucumber
- Eggplant
- Fructose
- Garbanzo beans (chickpeas)
- Grapefruit
- Green beans
- Hulless barley (lower GI than pearled)
- Lentils
- Lettuces
- Parsley
- Peaches (fresh)
- Peanuts*
- Pearled barley
- Plums
- Soybeans*
- Summer squashes

*under 20%

**These numbers fall into a range, so although both oranges and orange juice are listed, juices (no fiber) always have a higher GI than the fruits they come from; whole-wheat spaghetti has a lower GI than white-flour spaghetti.

PART FIVE

Exercise

Aerobic Walking

Brisk fitness walking—aerobic walking—is an exhilarating experience. Aerobic walking is one of the easiest and best forms of exercise for people with diabetes. It promotes overall health, proper blood circulation, and weight management. It is one of the best ways (along with weight training) to increase insulin sensitivity. Before beginning, invest in a pair of comfortable, supportive walking shoes. To avoid blisters, use "runners tape" (available in sporting goods stores) on your heels and toes.

Caution!

Exercise can lower blood sugar, and walking often has a profound effect on the body. People with diabetes should test their blood sugar level before and after exercise. Snacks or changes in medication might be needed if the exercise lowers your blood sugar.

Be sure to consult your doctor before starting any exercise program.

TO START OUT

If you are out of shape or not used to exercising, set small goals. Walk for five minutes a day until you feel comfortable walking more. Then increase your walking time to ten minutes, then to ten minutes twice a day. Be as consistent as you can. But most of all, never criticize yourself for not exercising and always praise yourself when you do! You want to start associating exercising with a feeling of success.

Eventually, you can set yourself a target of a twenty- to thirty-minute continuous brisk, invigorating walk. You can walk anywhere that is convenient and safe. Walk daily if you can. If not, walk every other day or as often as you can (even once a week to start).

At first, the easiest and quickest way to develop walking into a regular routine is to walk out your front door and do a circuit around your neighborhood. In the beginning, a neighborhood walk is recommended so that excuses (like "I don't have the time to go to the park or the nature trail") don't get in your way. ("I don't have time" is the number one excuse for not exercising.) You can walk anywhere that is convenient and safe.

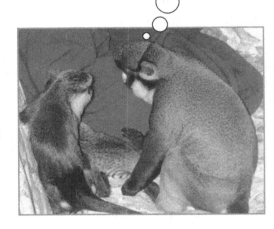

Your walking routine should suit your physical condition. If you have been inactive and are not used to physical exertion, start slowly: Walk for no more than twenty minutes every other day. Use a pace that challenges you but does not overtire you. Your goal is to exert yourself a little more each time until you reach a brisk pace that you feel comfortable with. In other words, you can gradually build up the duration and intensity of your routine until you reach your desired fitness level.

Avoid discouraging yourself by overdoing it in the beginning. Although walking is low impact (and therefore one of the safest forms of exercise), avoid the kind of exertion that leads to tired, aching, or swollen muscles and joints; leg cramps; and shin splints. If you cannot hold a conversation while you are walking without getting out of breath, you are walking too fast. Slow down. Also, if you feel any pain in your legs, slow down. At the end of your walk, you should feel refreshed. If you feel tired, you are walking too fast.

HEART RATE

Your resting heart rate (pulse rate) is a measure of your state of well-being. Pulse rates vary. Low pulse rates are common in people who take drugs known as beta-blockers. Generally, the lower the resting pulse rate, the healthier you are. The average rate for men is between 70 and 85 beats per minute; the average rate for women tends to be faster and is between 75 and 90 beats per minute.

Take your pulse rate first thing in the morning, before it has had time to be increased by exertion, mental excitement, foods, or caffeinated drinks. Sit quietly and breathe normally. Place the first two fingers of your right hand on the main artery of the inner wrist of your left hand just below the base of the thumb. Count the number of beats in a fifteen-second interval and multiply the number of beats by four to get your resting pulse rate.

Aerobic Walking Pulse Rate

To get the benefits of aerobic walking, you have to achieve a walking pulse rate between 60 percent and 85 percent of your maximum heart rate. There is a simple way to calculate your aerobic walking pulse rate. (This formula gives you an average number that works for most people.) Subtract your age from 220. This gives you your maximum heart rate in beats per minute. Next, multiply your maximum heart rate by 0.60 (60 percent) for the lower end of your aerobic walking pulse rate and by 0.85 (85 percent) for the higher end. The table below has done the calculations for you for ages in multiples of ten. For kids under the age of fifteen, an average aerobic heart rate range is 165 to 175.

Age	Max. Heart Rate	60% Level	85% Level
20	200	120	170
25	195	117	166
30	190	114	162
35	185	111	157
40	180	108	153
45	175	105	149
50	170	102	145
55	165	99	140

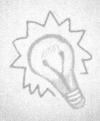

A Good Idea!

Here's an easy way to determine if you are exercising within your aerobic heart rate range:

1. If your breathing is comfortable and talking is easy, you are probably below your aerobic range.

2. If breathing is deep and speaking is possible, you are exercising in your range.

3. Gasping or being unable to speak more than three words together are signs that you are over your aerobic range.

To double-check the formulas, after you have been walking for about ten minutes, stop and take your pulse. Be sure to have a watch with you that records seconds. Take your pulse the same way you calculated your resting pulse rate as explained above. If your heart is beating beyond the high end of your aerobic range (85 percent), you are walking too fast. When you first start out you should stick to the lower end of your aerobic range (60 percent) until you feel comfortable with it. Then, as you progress, measure your aerobic improvement by taking your pulse at several points during the walk and immediately upon finishing. This will ensure that you remain within your aerobic range. As your fitness improves, you will find that your heart rate decreases while performing the same level of exercise. This is because the increased size and strength of the heart muscle enables it to pump a larger volume of blood into the arteries with each beat. Once you are comfortable walking at the 60 percent level, experiment up to the 70 to 75 percent level. You should not need to go higher than this. At this level, you should get all the benefits that you need.

WALKING TECHNIQUE

With proper technique, aerobic walking is one of the safest and most beneficial forms of exercise and a terrific way to lose weight. Walking should be a very fluid movement that is easy on the body. Warm up with stretches before you start.

To develop a good stride, start with good posture. Your spine should be straight, tall, and relaxed. Don't put an unnatural arch in your lower back. This can create great discomfort, especially when walking long distances.

Keep your chest up, relax your shoulders, and swing your arms, with your elbows bent at ninety-degree angles, naturally with each step. Straight arms on long walks can lead to swelling, tingling, and numbness of the fingers or hands. Bent arms eliminates this and will help you gain upper body strength and toning of your deltoids, biceps, and triceps. Also, by bending your arms, you will burn 5 to 10 percent more calories. One more great reason to keep your arms bent and swinging in a fluid motion is that it will help you pick up your pace for longer periods of time. Your hands should be relaxed and slightly cupped.

Walking uses the abdominal muscles and hip flexors. The hip flexors rotate the hip forward and lead the leg in its forward motion.

Push off from your toes and balls of your feet. Your feet should land firmly on ground, striking from heel to toe. As one leg swings forward and straightens, your body will land easily on the heel. Your ankle should be flexed with your toes pointed upward at about a forty-five degree angle from the ground. The foot placement should be in front of the body, as if almost walking along a straight line. (The shortest distance between two points is a straight line.) As the body's weight passes over the leading leg, the foot should roll forward and push off from the toes to begin the next step. A strong push will give you more momentum and power. As you practice stepping and increase your hip flexibility, you will naturally develop a slightly longer stride.

Do not bend forward while walking. This is the most common mistake among walkers and may lead to lower back, leg, foot, hip, and neck problems. It is also potentially harmful to your back if you try to increase the length of your stride by taking longer unnatural steps. Speed and efficiency in walking are generated by hip flexibility and quicker, not longer, steps.

For additional information on walking and aerobic exercise, read exercise physiologist Covert Baily's timeless classic *Fit or Fat* (Houghton Mifflin Company, 1978).

Weight-Resistance Training

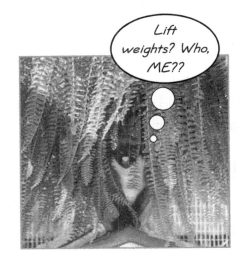

Lift weights? Who, ME??

These easy exercises are to STRENGTHEN your muscles! You can do weight-resistance training in your own living room while listening to music or watching TV! Check with your doctor before doing weight-resistance training because it can affect the blood sugar levels of someone with diabetes. You will probably need a snack before weight lifting and one after.

Wear comfortable clothes. Have water on hand to keep from becoming dehydrated. Warm up by stretching or doing aerobics before you weight train.

Choose dumbbells that allow you to complete twelve repetitions (leaving you too tired for a thirteenth). This challenges your muscles so you will have better results in gaining strength. If you are a beginner, start with two- or three-pound weights and buy heavier ones as you progress.

Twelve repetitions (reps) equals one set. Do three to four sets of each exercise. For example, twelve crunches is one set; rest for a minute or so, then do another set. If you can't do that many, start with two or three as a set—or however many you can do! When first starting, consider using a mirror to check your positioning. You can also hire a personal trainer to give you tips and motivation!

Exercise two different muscle groups each day. By working different muscle groups each day, by the end of the week, you will have worked all of your muscle groups (with extra emphasis on the abs). As you advance, you can add more weight to the weight-resistance exercises or add more repetitions.

Exercise is more effective when you concentrate on the muscle you are exercising at the time!

Weight lifting (weight-resistance training) is generally recommended for people aged twelve and over. (Sports, such as basketball, are recommended to promote muscle toning for people age 12 and under.) Weight lifting is especially helpful to people with type 2 diabetes. It is helpful in decreasing insulin resistance.

The daily exercises shown in this section (two exercises for each day of the week) will take less than ten minutes a day.

If you don't have a set of weights, find other easy-to-hold items to lift, such as food cans or water bottles.

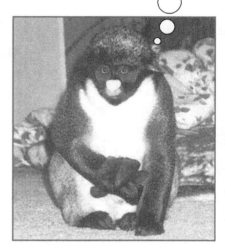

Okay. I'll do ten reps with my little bear.

DAY 1

Thighs, Back of: Hamstrings

Lie with your front side on the floor, resting your chin on your forearms on the floor; exhale while curling your legs up. Hold for one second and inhale as you lower your feet back to the floor. Use ankle weights for more resistance.

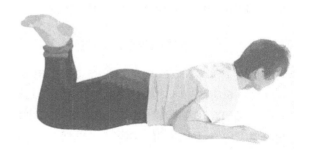

Thighs, Front of: Squats

Stand with your feet slightly wider than your shoulders and your arms at your sides. Exhale as you squat slowly, bending your knees and pushing your rear end out. Keep your back straight, abs tight, and don't let your knees go past your toes. Squeeze your thighs and glutes for added contraction. At the same time,

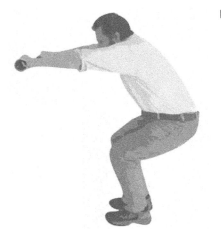

raise your arms straight in front of you until they're extended straight out at shoulder height, palms facing each other. Hold for one second, then inhale as you stand back up. Don't lock your knees when you return to standing. Hold dumbbells for more resistance.

DAY 2

Shoulders: Side Raises

Stand with your feet shoulder-width apart. Hold a dumbbell in each hand, arms at your sides and palms toward your body. Keeping your arms straight, your back straight, and your palms turned downward, lift the weights up to chin level and hold for one second. Lower them back slowly to starting position.

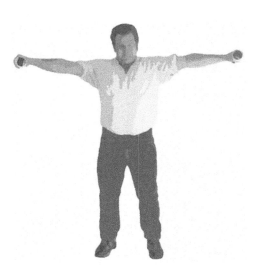

Abs (Stomach): Crunches

Lie on the floor with your knees bent and feet flat on the floor. Bend your elbows out to the sides of your head, fingers touching your ears. Keep a tennis ball's distance between your chin and chest. Keep your lower back pressed to the floor as you curl your upper body forward and up. Don't pull on your neck when you come up. Hold the highest position for one second before lowering back to the floor, slowly and with control. Return to a point where your upper body is just off the floor and your abs are still contracted.

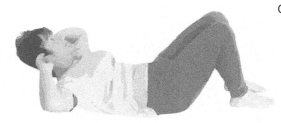

DAY 3

Chest: Chest Press

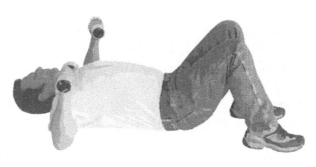

Lie on a workout bench or on the floor. Keeping your head flat on the floor, raise your arms over your head, shoulder-width apart, palms facing toward your knees, so that the dumbbells are positioned right over your collarbones, end to end. Bend your elbows ninety degrees, slowly lowering the weights until your elbows touch the floor. With control, push the dumbbells back up to the staring position.

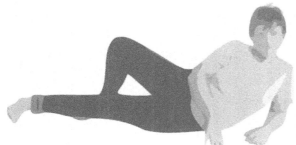

Thighs, Inner: Inner Thigh Leg Raises

Lying on the floor, bend your right knee and place your right foot behind your left leg. Keep your left leg straight as you exhale slowly and lift the left foot as high as you can. Hold for one second; inhale as you lower, slowly and with control. Repeat on the opposite side for one rep. Use ankle weights for more resistance.

DAY 4

Calves: Angled Calf Raises

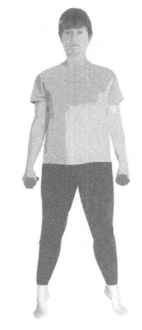

Stand with feet shoulder-width apart, as you hold a dumb-bell in each hand; turn your feet out to form a forty-five-degree angle. Exhale as you rise up onto your toes. Keep your chest lifted, shoulders back, and abs tight. Hold for one second and inhale as you lower back down. Hold dumbbells at your sides for more resistance.

Glutes: Glute Squeeze

Lie on the floor on your back with palms
flat on the floor; exhale as you lift your
pelvis three to six inches off the floor.
Squeeze your buttock muscles for
one second, then inhale as you
lower back down.

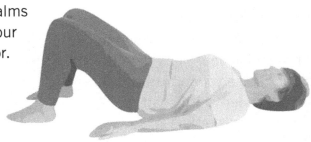

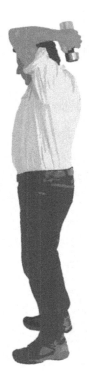

DAY 5

Arms, Back of (Triceps): Dumbbell Extensions

Hold a dumbbell in each hand and raise your arms straight
above your head, keeping elbows close to the head and
slightly bent. Inhale as you lower the dumbbell behind your
head with control as shown. Hold for one second and exhale
as you raise your arms slowly and with control.

Thighs, Outer: Outer Thigh Leg Raises

Get on your knees with your hands on the floor, keeping your
back straight and head up; exhale as you raise your bent leg
out to the side. Hold for one second and inhale as you lower
your leg. Switch sides for one rep. Use ankle weights for
more resistance.

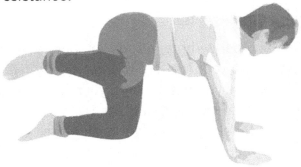

DAY 6

Back: Alternate Limb Back Builders

From a position of "all fours" on
the floor, exhale and extend
your right arm and left
leg. Balance on your
right knee and hold for
three seconds. Exhale as you
lower your arm and leg. Repeat
on the opposite side for one rep.

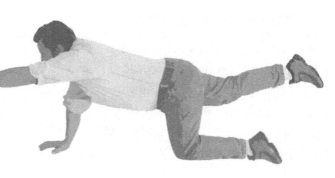

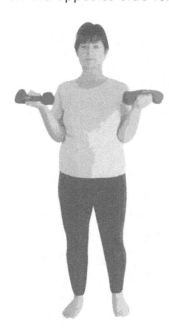

Arms, Front of (Biceps): Standing Dumbbell Curls

Hold a weight in each hand, palms facing up, elbows
bent and relaxed at your sides. Exhale when you curl
your arms up toward your shoulders. Keep your wrists
straight and hold your arms just above a ninety-degree
angle for one second, as shown. Exhale and lower your
arms slowly and with control.

DAY 7

Day 7 is optional. It can be a day of rest or
you can do these two extra ab exercises!

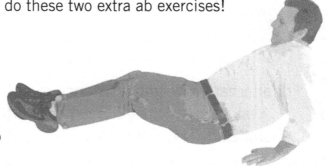

Abs (Stomach): Bent Knee Ab Crunches

Sit with heels above the floor;
exhale as you slowly bring your
heels and knees toward your torso

until your thighs and knees make a ninety-degree angle. Hold for one second. Exhale as you extend your legs back out, slowly and with control.

Abs (Stomach): Twist Crunches

Lie on the floor with your knees bent and the side of your lower foot on the floor. Let your legs fall as far as they can to your left side, leaving your upper body flat on the floor and your lower body on its

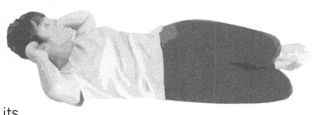

side. Bend your elbows out to the sides of your head, fingers touching your ears. Keep a tennis ball's distance between your chin and chest. Keep your lower back pressed to the floor as you curl your upper body forward and slightly up. Don't pull on your neck when you come up. Hold the highest position for one second before lowering back to the floor. Concentrate on contracting the muscles on the sides of your waist (the obliques). Complete your number of reps on one side and switch to the other.

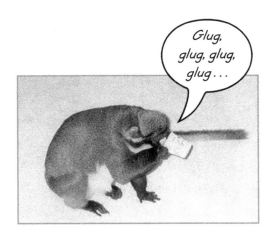

Glug, glug, glug, glug . . .

P.S. Don't forget to drink your water when you're done weight training!

For alternative weight-resistance exercises, visit Molly's website at **www.hellomolly.com**. For additional information, read *Body For Life* by Bill Phillips (HarperCollins, 1999).

Terms to Know

adult-onset diabetes. Former term for non–insulin-dependent or type 2 diabetes.

aerobic exercise. Any steady physical exercise, such as bicycling, swimming, and running, that makes the heart and lungs work harder (bringing the heart rate up) to meet the muscles' need for oxygen.

alpha cells. A type of cell in the pancreas (in areas called the islets of Langerhans); alpha cells make and release a hormone called glucagon, which raises the level of glucose (blood sugar) in the blood.

alternative therapies. Treatments that are considered to be outside the mainstream of medical practice, including nutritional supplementation, relaxation therapy, prayer, imagery and visualization, meditation, massage, and music therapy.

amino acids. The building blocks of protein. Some amino acids are recommended as supplements for people with diabetes.

antidiabetic agent. A substance that helps a person with diabetes to control the level of glucose in the blood.

antioxidants. Compounds that minimize the oxidation of tissues. They also help control free-radical damage.

artificial pancreas. A large machine used in hospitals that constantly measures glucose in the blood and, in response, releases the right amount of insulin. (Research scientists are working to develop a small unit to be implanted in the body, which would function like a real pancreas.)

beta cells. Pancreatic islet cells that secrete insulin.

blood sugar. See **glucose**.

blood sugar meter. A handheld machine that tests blood sugar levels.

brittle diabetes. A condition characterized by extreme fluctuations in blood sugar levels within a short period of time. Occurs in a small percentage of type 1 patients, especially after the first year. Also called labile or unstable diabetes.

calories. Units representing the amount of energy provided by food. Carbohydrate, protein, and fat are the primary sources of calories in the diet.

carbohydrate. One of three major sources of calories in the diet. Carbohydrates are chains of sugar molecules hooked together. Carbohydrate is broken down into glucose during digestion and is the main nutrient that raises blood sugar levels.

cholesterol. A type of fat that comes in the form of "good" (HDL) cholesterol and "bad" (LDL) cholesterol.

diabetes mellitus. Diabetes. A metabolic disease in which the body cannot get energy from glucose in the normal way, either because the body doesn't make enough insulin or cannot use the insulin it has. The metabolism of carbohydrates, proteins, and fats is altered. There are several forms of diabetes mellitus, including insulin-dependent diabetes mellitus (IDDM or type 1), non–insulin-dependent diabetes mellitus (NIDDM or type 2), and gestational diabetes mellitus.

diabetes pills. Pills or capsules that are taken by mouth to lower the blood glucose level by increasing insulin production or by helping the body to use insulin properly or by decreasing sugar production and absorption.

diabetic coma. A severe emergency in which a person loses consciousness due to blood sugar (glucose) levels that are either too low or too high. If the glucose level is too low, the person has hypoglycemia; if the level is too high, the person has hyperglycemia and may develop ketoacidosis. Also see **hyperglycemia, hypoglycemia,** and **ketoacidosis.**

diabetic eye disease. A disease of the small blood vessels of the retina of the eye in people with diabetes. In this disease, the vessels swell and leak liquid into the retina, blurring vision and sometimes leading to blindness.

diabetic neuropathy. Temporary or permanent damage to nerve tissue. Injury to the nerves is caused by decreased blood flow and high blood sugar levels. Neuropathies are more likely to develop if blood glucose levels are poorly controlled.

Edmonton protocol. A method developed at the University of Alberta in Edmonton for transplanting healthy islets from a donor to replace missing islets in patients with type 1 diabetes. The method requires the use of immunosupressive drugs to prevent rejection of the transplanted islets. Because of the undesirable side effects of these drugs, use of the procedure is restricted to patients with hypoglycemia unawareness, for whom the risks posed by the drugs can be justified.

essential fatty acids (EFAs). "Good" fats not made by the body that must be obtained from food for the proper functioning of the body. Fatty acids provide the raw materials that help in the control of blood pressure, blood clotting, inflammation, hormone production, and other important body functions.

fasting plasma glucose test. A diagnostic test for diabetes, performed after the patient has had nothing to eat or drink overnight.

fat. The most concentrated source of energy in foods. Fat is a nutrient that is an important source of calories; one gram of fat supplies 9 calories, more than twice the amount we get from protein or carbohydrates. About 10 percent of the fat we eat can be converted to glucose in the body.

fiber. A type of carbohydrate; sometimes called roughage or bulk. Fiber is the part of plants that the body does not break down during digestion. Adequate fiber intake keeps the digestive tract working smoothly.

gestational diabetes. A condition in which high blood sugar levels develop during pregnancy in women who were not previously diabetic. Diagnosed at twenty-four to twenty-eight weeks gestation. Levels usually return to normal after delivery, but about 50 percent of mothers with gestational diabetes later develop type 2 diabetes.

glucagon. A hormone produced by the alpha cells of the pancreas; increases blood sugar levels.

glucagon kit. An emergency kit containing a pre-mixed form of the hormone, used in treating hypoglycemic episodes in unconscious diabetic patients.

glucose. Blood sugar; a simple sugar obtained from the breakdown of carbohydrates in food; the body's source of quick energy after a meal.

glycemic index (GI). A way of classifying carbohydrate foods we eat (such as rice, cereal, potato, or pasta) according to their effect on blood sugar.

glycogen. The form in which glucose is stored in the liver and muscles.

healthcare team. The group of healthcare professionals who help a patient manage diabetes. This team may include a physician, registered dietitian, and certified diabetes educator (a certified diabetes educator can also be a physician, registered nurse, or registered dietitian). Ophthalmologists, podiatrists, and other specialists can also be part of the team.

high blood glucose. A condition that occurs in people with diabetes when their blood glucose levels are too high. Symptoms include urinating often, being very thirsty, and losing weight. Also called hyperglycemia.

honeymoon phase. A temporary remission that occurs in about 20 percent of type 1 patients shortly after the onset of diabetes. Pancreatic insulin secretion resumes to some degree, but usually only for a few weeks or months.

hyperglycemia. See **high blood glucose**.

hyperinsulinemia. A condition in which the pancreas produces too much insulin, which results in too much insulin in the bloodstream.

hypermolar syndrome. The result of chronically very high blood sugar levels (blood sugar levels so high that the blood thickens) and dehydration. Hypermolar syndrome usually occurs in older people with type 2 diabetes. Ketones are not present. Symptoms include tiredness, confusion, and coma. Hypermolar syndrome may be brought on in people with type 2 diabetes by stress related to a major illness or by taking steroids.

hypoglycemia. See **low blood sugar**.

hypoglycemia unawareness. A dangerous condition in which the patient does not experience the usual warning signs of low blood sugar.

hypoglycemic reaction. A group of symptoms that occur when blood sugar levels drop too low (below about 50 mg/dL) in a person with diabetes. The reaction is caused by too much insulin, too much exercise, too little food, or other factors.

impaired glucose tolerance. A term used to describe blood glucose levels falling between normal and diabetic range; not considered a form of diabetes but a precursor to development of diabetes, if ignored.

inject. To force a liquid into the body with a needle and syringe.

insulin. A hormone produced in the pancreas. Helps glucose enter the body cells, where it is used for energy.

insulin pen. A small, pre-filled pen-shaped device with a sharp, disposable needle; used to inject insulin.

insulin pump. A mechanical pump for continuous insulin delivery. It is lightweight and small and can be worn on a belt or in a pocket. Pumps deliver insulin continuously through a needle inserted under the skin near the abdomen.

insulin resistance. Linked to type 2 diabetes, resistance of the body cells to take in glucose even in the presence of insulin. Insulin resistance occurs when there is plenty of insulin made by the pancreas (amounts can be even higher than what a normal pancreas makes), but the cells of the body have become resistant or insensitive to the action of insulin.

intensive insulin regimen. The use of multiple daily insulin injections or an insulin infusion pump to achieve tight control of blood sugar level; administration of insulin and frequent self-monitoring of blood glucose.

islet transplantation. Transplanting healthy islets from a donor into a person with type 1 diabetes to replace missing islets. (Visit www.isletmedical.com for more information on islet transplantation.)

islets of Langerhans. Clusters of cells in the pancreas; the islets contain beta cells, alpha cells, and delta cells.

jet injector. A needle-free device that projects insulin through the skin under high pressure.

ketoacidosis. A dangerous condition in which ketone levels build up in the blood and ketones "spill" into the urine. Diabetic ketoacidosis occurs when the body is so low in insulin, it starts using stored fat as fuel. Ketones are a byproduct of the fat breaking down. Large quantities of ketones cause the body to become overly acidic. Diabetic ketoacidosis is a medical emergency. Symptoms include nausea, breathing difficulty, sweet-smelling breath, confusion, and coma.

ketones (ketone bodies). Waste products produced when fatty acids are broken down for energy.

ketonuria. The presence of ketones in the urine.

lancet. A small, sharp device for making a small incision in the skin.

lasette. A portable, battery-operated laser that pricks the skin as easily and accurately as lancets. (Available by prescription only.)

low blood sugar. A condition that occurs in people with diabetes when their blood glucose levels are too low. Symptoms include feeling anxious or confused, feeling numb in the arms and hands, and shaking or feeling dizzy. Also called hypoglycemia.

meal plan. A guide to help people get the proper amount of calories, carbohydrates, proteins, fats, vitamins, minerals, and fiber in their diet.

minerals. Inorganic elements, such as calcium, iron, potassium, sodium, zinc, or chromium, that are essential to the nutrition of humans, animals, and plants. Deficiencies of certain minerals are thought to contribute to diabetes.

non–insulin-dependent diabetes. See **type 2 diabetes.**

obesity. An increase in body weight caused by excessive accumulation of fat.

oral glucose tolerance test (OGTT). A (rarely necessary) diagnostic test for diabetes. The patient fasts overnight and several blood samples are drawn the next morning (over a two-hour period) after the patient drinks a sugary drink.

oral hypoglycemic drugs. Drugs taken by mouth by some patients with type 2 diabetes to help lower blood sugar levels. These drugs do not contain insulin, but improve insulin action in the body.

pancreas. A gland behind the stomach; contains clusters of cells including beta cells, which secrete insulin. Also secretes digestive enzymes into the small intestine.

polydipsia. Excessive thirst.

polyols. Substances that accumulate in the lens of the eye and eventually cause damage to the lens. Polyols are caused by elevated glucose levels in the lens of the eye.

polyphagia. Excessive appetite or overeating.

polyuria. Frequent urination.

protein. One of the three major sources of calories in the diet. Protein is made of chains of amino acids. Those with "essential amino acids" (amino acids the body cannot make) are known as "complete proteins." Up to 50 percent of protein consumed is converted by the liver into glycogen. The rest is used for growth, repair of cells and tissues, and other functions.

random plasma glucose test. A diagnostic test for diabetes; performed without concern for the time of the most recent meal.

renal threshold. The blood sugar level at which the kidneys "spill" excess sugar from the blood into the urine; the average is about 180 mg/dL, but wide variation exists.

risk factors. Traits that make it more likely that a person will get an illness. For example, a risk factor for getting diabetes is having a family history of diabetes.

secondary diabetes. A condition in which the pancreas or another organ is damaged by disease, chemicals, or drugs, causing interference with insulin production.

self-monitoring of blood glucose (SMBG). A method for people with diabetes to find out how much glucose is in their blood. A drop of blood from the fingertip is placed on a special coated strip of paper that "reads" (through an electronic meter) the amount of glucose in the blood.

supplements. Preparations (pills, tablets, or powders) taken to supply nutrients.

type 1 diabetes. An autoimmune disorder, the type of diabetes in which the pancreas produces no insulin or extremely small amounts. People with type 1 diabetes need to take insulin injections in order to live.

type 2 diabetes. The type of diabetes in which the body doesn't use its insulin effectively (insulin resistance) and/or doesn't produce enough insulin.

unit of insulin. The basic measure of insulin. U-100 insulin means 100 units of insulin per milliliter (mL) or cubic centimeter (cc) of solution. Most insulin made today in the United States is U-100.

unstable diabetes. A type of diabetes in which a person's blood sugar level often swings quickly from high to low and from low to high. Also called "brittle diabetes" or "labile diabetes."

vitamins. Any of various fat-soluble or water-soluble calorie-free organic substances, essential in small amounts for normal growth and activity of the body.

weight lifting. Also called "resistance exercise"; a form of exercise in which you use the muscles in your body to resist the motion of some other force (coming from your own body weight, hand-held dumbbells or weight-resistance training machines); shown to improve insulin resistance in people with type 2 diabetes.

yeast infection. An infection that is usually caused by a fungus; yeast infections occur more frequently in women with diabetes. Symptoms can include itching, burning when urinating, pain, and vaginal discharge.

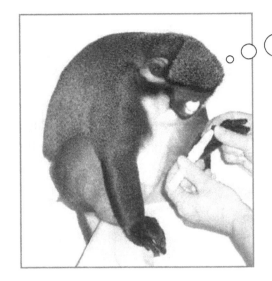

Taking good care of yourself just takes a little extra time.

I have plenty of time left over for hanging out and having fun!

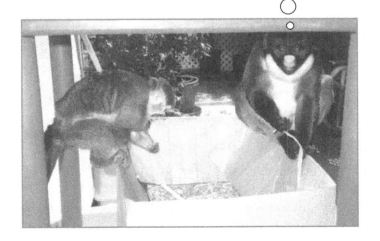

Suggested Reading

The Carbohydrate Addict's Healthy Heart Program by Richard F. Heller, M.D., Rachael F. Heller, M.D., and Frederic J. Vagnini, M.D. (New York, NY: Ballantine Publishing Group, 1999).

Dr. Atkins Vita-Nutrient Solution by Robert C. Atkins, M.D. (New York, NY: Fireside, 1998).

Fats That Heal, Fats That Kill by Udo Erasmus, Ph.D. (Burnaby BC, Canada: Alive Books, 1993).

Enter The Zone by Barry Sears, Ph.D. (New York, NY: HarperCollins, 1995).

Nutrition Made Simple by Robert Crayhon, Ph.D. (New York, NY: M Evans & Co., 1996).

Nutritionally Incorrect, 2nd edition, by Allan Spreen, M.D. (Pleasant Grove, UT: Woodland Publishing, 2001).

The Protein Power Life Plan by Michael Eades, M.D., and Mary Dan Eades, M.D. (New York, NY: Warner Books, 2001).

The Schwarzbein Principle by Diana Schwarzbein, M.D., and Nancy Deville (Deerfield Beach, FL: Health Communications, 1999.)

For additional support and information on diabetes,
including many useful links,
visit Molly's website at **www.hellomolly.com**.

Index